HEALTH CARE RIGHTS

Other Avon Books by
Nancy Levitin

RETIREMENT RIGHTS

HEALTH CARE RIGHTS

NANCY LEVITIN, ESQ.

AVON BOOKS ◆ NEW YORK

This publication is not engaged in rendering medical, legal, accounting, or other professional services. If medical, legal, or other expert assistance is required, the services of a competent professional should be sought.

AVON BOOKS
A division of
The Hearst Corporation
1350 Avenue of the Americas
New York, New York 10019

Copyright © 1996 by Nancy Levitin
Published by arrangement with the author
Library of Congress Catalog Card Number: 95-49196
ISBN: 0-380-78025-9

Library of Congress Cataloging in Publication Data:

Levitin, Nancy.
   Health care rights / Nancy Levitin.
      p.   cm.
Includes bibliographical references and index.
1. Patients—Legal status, laws, etc.—United States—Popular works.   2. Medical care—Law and legislation—United States—Popular works.   I. Title.
KF3823.Z9L48   1996   95-49196
344.73'041—dc20   CIP
[347.30441]

First Avon Book Trade Printing: June 1996

AVON TRADEMARK REG. U.S. PAT. OFF. AND IN OTHER COUNTRIES, MARCA REGISTRADA, HECHO EN U.S.A.

Printed in the U.S.A.

Q   10 9 8 7 6 5 4 3 2 1

To Mitch—you made it possible

Contents

Introduction

I had written about 25 percent of this book when I had an epiphany. If the year were 1986 instead of 1996, I'd be done already! Health care rights are a relatively new phenomenon. Most of the judicial decisions and legislative enactments that protect the rights of health care consumers today did not exist a decade ago.

The push for health care reform ushered in with the Clinton administration dramatically impacted our heath care rights. Take, for example, the rights of patients who have been injured at the hands of incompetent doctors. People started asking questions about whether these patients should continue to have a right to recover whatever amount of damages a jury awards them, or whether malpractice awards should be capped to control health care spending. New concerns were voiced about the rights of patients who belong to managed care plans, such as HMOs. What rights, if any, should these patients have to receive the "best" care if the "best" doctors do not belong to their HMO's network of providers? Our right to quality health care and compensation for medical malpractice are covered in chapter 1.

Recent advances in medical technology have complicated our right to give or withhold our consent to a proposed treatment. We are now confronted with confounding medical choices that did not exist a few years ago. Our doctors are asking us to decide what should be done with a fetus after sophisticated prenatal testing reveals a serious congenital disorder. When we are diagnosed with an illness, we must elect from a perplexing array of treatment options including organ transplants, microscopic surgery, and aggressive medication regimens. We are offered information about our precise life expectancy and genetic predisposition to chronic or fatal illnesses. Do we have a right to this information? Do we even *want* this information? Informed consent is the subject of chapter 2.

Our entry into the computer age has posed new threats to the privacy of our medical records. Can large data banks of patient information be adequately protected against security breaches? What about medical records sent by fax between doctors and hospitals? With the AIDS epidemic in full bloom, risks associated with informational piracy have assumed a new dimension of seriousness. The stigmatizing and devastating nature of this illness has made us more fearful than ever that information about our health will fall into the wrong hands. Chapter 3 covers our right to privacy in medical matters.

Before President Bush signed the Omnibus Budget Reconciliation Act into law on December 19, 1989, hospitals receiving Medicare payments were not required to comply with the federal "anti-dumping act." The anti-dumping act prohibits hospital emergency rooms from "dumping" poor and uninsured patients out the door without proper care. Chapter 4 looks at the rights of hospitalized patients and suggests ways you can protect your interests, from the moment you learn you may need to enter the hospital through your discharge.

Not until 1987 did the federal government pass comprehensive legislation setting standards of care for nursing home residents. Now the access of nursing home residents to nutritious food, high-quality rehabilitation services, respectful and courteous treatment, and restraint-free care are federally regulated. In chapter 5, the new and old rights of nursing home residents are covered, as well as advocacy tips for residents' friends and family.

In 1990 the U.S. Supreme Court first articulated our constitutional right to control our health care after the onset of incapacity. Congress took action one year later when it passed the Patient Self-Determination Act. Today every state in the nation gives its residents the right to set forth their health care wishes in an advance medical directive. Our right to control our medical treatment through the use of living wills, health care powers of attorney, and state surrogate decision-making laws is examined in chapter 6.

Judicial challenges to statutory bans on assisted suicide only began to sprout up across the country in the early 1990s. About the same time, many state legislatures started debating whether to allow doctors to help their terminally ill patients die. Meanwhile, the medical profession grappled with the ethical implications of physician-assisted suicide as two of their own revealed the role they had played in helping seriously ill patients end their lives. The troubling issues of assisted suicide and euthanasia are explored in chapter 7.

Our health is perhaps our greatest vulnerability. When we lose our good health, our independence, strength, and confidence are also thrown into jeopardy. We are fortunate that laws have recently been passed, and judicial decisions rendered, to protect us in times of illness, when we are most exposed. Now we must assume responsibility for educating ourselves about our health care rights and for safeguarding those rights from abuse. This book provides the information we need to become informed health care advocates for ourselves and our loved ones.

The second edition of this book, if and when it is published ten years from now, will be twice as long as this book if our health care rights continue to multiply at the same prodigious rate.

ONE

Your Right to Quality Medical Care

You've read the headlines in the newspaper: "Surgeon Removes Patient's Healthy Kidney by Mistake"; "Eight-year-old Dies During Routine Ear Operation"; "Thousands of Hysterectomies Found to be Unnecessary."

To those of us who have been raised to revere doctors, these stories are particularly disturbing and disillusioning. We *want* to be able to turn ourselves over, body and soul, to the healing hands of our doctors. We resist words admonishing us to ask our doctors lots of questions and become educated health care consumers. The image of an all-trustworthy physician is too alluring.

On some level, however, even the most self-deluded of us recognize that doctors are only human. As such, they are capable of human error.

Human error is just human error, except when the person doing the erring is a doctor. Then the stakes are infinitely higher. Doctors are uniquely qualified to both assist in miraculous cures and leave unspeakable emotional and physical pain in the wake of their mistakes.

What patients are at greatest risk of becoming victims of medical malpractice? Is there anything you can do to minimize your exposure to negligent practitioners? The first section of this chapter considers some examples of medical malpractice and offers tips for selecting qualified health care providers.

The second section of the chapter takes a look at the current system of policing the medical profession. Does the existing array of public agencies, private watchdog organizations, and professional associations succeed at ridding the medical profession of bad apples?

Medical malpractice litigation itself is the subject of the third section of the chapter. Which patients decide to sue their providers, and why? What must an injured patient prove in order to prevail against a medical professional who allegedly provided substandard care? How do plaintiffs' attorneys help their clients win sizable awards?

Alternatives to malpractice litigation are covered in the fourth and final section of the chapter. Bringing and defending a lawsuit takes an emotional and financial toll on plaintiffs and defendants alike. Can the system be reformed to make the process quicker and cheaper? Are there any less costly ways for doctors and patients to resolve their differences?

THE MEDICAL MALPRACTICE RISK

Lawyers who are accused of driving up the cost of health care in their pursuit of the almighty malpractice dollar have these words of advice for their critics: Redirect your line of fire. Affix your guns on the medical profession.

Medical malpractice poses a real risk to each and every one of us. According to a 1992 Harvard medical practice study, 27,000 "negligent adverse events" occurred in one year in New York State hospitals alone. Seven thousand of these events resulted in a patient's death, and almost 1,000 resulted in permanent disability.[1]

Numbers like these lend credibility to charges that the medical profession is unable to maintain high standards of care within its ranks. As long as doctors continue to provide their patients with substandard care, society will have to bear the financial and nonfinancial costs of malpractice.

Every patient must recognize the risks that attend even the most frequently performed medical procedures. The discussion that follows looks at two hotbeds of malpractice—the practices of prescribing medications, and treating illnesses that afflict women exclusively or primarily. At least half of us have been exposed to one or both of these medical practices. Included in the discussion is a look at how computers have begun to protect us from our doctors' all-too-human frailties in these two areas.

The second part of the section offers some tips for picking quality doctors, hospitals, and Health Maintenance Organizations (HMOs).

MEDICATION ERRORS

Even the bravest of souls may entertain fleeting doubts about her surgeon's competency as she is wheeled into the operating room and the mask of oblivion is positioned over her face. How many patients worry, though, when their doctor takes out his or her prescription pad? What about when the pharmacist hands over a bag containing a new prescription drug? Are these occasions for concern?

They should be. Medication errors are the second most common cause of lawsuits against doctors, according to a Physician Insurers Association of America (PIAA) study. Over 42 percent of medication errors studied involved significant permanent injuries, including death.[2]

The most frequently lodged medication-related complaint alleged by patients is that the doctor prescribed the incorrect dosage. Incorrect dosages can result in permanent damage to the central nervous system, anaphylaxis (a rare, severe, and life-threatening allergic reaction), respiratory failure, gastrointestinal bleeding, other injuries, and death.

Inappropriate prescriptions underlie the second most common medication-related malpractice claim. Doctors that get the dosage right have been sued for prescribing a medication that is not an appropriate treatment of the patient's medical ailment.

Doctors who prescribe the right dose of the right medication can still be sued for prescribing a drug that is not appropriate for a particular patient. Patients who have an allergic reaction to an otherwise correctly prescribed medication also file medication-related malpractice claims against their doctors.

Take, for example, a doctor who prescribes one of the four drug classes most likely to trigger allergic reactions in patients: an antibiotic; a non-steroidal anti-inflammatory; an anticonvulsant; or a diuretic. When taking the patient's medical history, the doctor inquires "Any allergies?" The patient responds in the negative. Later the patient suffers an allergic reaction to the medication and sues for malpractice. She alleges that the doctor acted negligently in not specifically questioning her about allergies to the particular medication being prescribed, given the enhanced risk of an allergic reaction to that specific drug.

Finally, patients file medication-related malpractice claims when their doctors fail to monitor drug usage, effects, or side effects, when they neglect to read the patient's medical records before dispensing the medication, or when they fail to warn their patients of the possibility of becoming addicted to the prescribed drug.

If you have been injured as a result of a prescription medication, review the discussions you had with the prescribing physician. To what extent did the doctor discuss the medication with you? Did he or she explain possible side effects of the drug? Review the benefits and drawbacks of alternative medications and treatment options? Question you about other drugs you are taking, both prescribed and over-the-counter? Inquire into known allergies? Provide you with any written material? Ask you to repeat back the information provided to you?

Doctors that are best protected against malpractice prescribe the least toxic drug available to meet the patient's needs, explain to the patient all of the risks, benefits, and side effects associated with the drug, solicit questions and provide complete answers, document their discussions with copious notes, and distribute written instructional material. Written materials are especially important when the instructions for taking the drug are complicated. Patients should not be expected to remember to take the drug on a full stomach every four hours, avoid aspirin, schedule monthly follow-up exams, *and* be on the lookout for a quarter-sized rash with raised pimples that may form on the inside of the left thigh in a month.

Patients harmed by prescription medications may, however, be at least partially responsible for causing their own injuries. A patient who mixes a prescription medication with alcohol, for example, probably bears some responsibility for the injuries that result if the prescribing doctor expressly warned the patient about the risks of drinking while medicated. Patients who share responsibility with their doctors for medication-related injuries are said to have contributory negligence. A finding of contributory negligence in a malpractice action can reduce or eliminate the damages available to the injured patient-plaintiff.

A coauthor of the PIAA study concluded that many of the injuries the researchers found resulting from prescription medications could have been avoided. A second study conducted by researchers at two large Boston hospitals similarly found that more than 40 percent of the most serious drug reactions in hospitals caused by doctors' and nurses' mistakes might have been preventable.[3] Drug malpractice, by and large, results from physician ignorance, laziness, or poor doctor-patient communication.

Computers can help improve the medical profession's medication malpractice track record. On the market today are several medication databases that list upwards of 5,000 drugs, with indications, contraindications, and correct dosages. Drug interaction programs identify risks associated with combining prescription and nonprescription drugs. Computer-generated patient instruction sheets explain the purpose of the drug, when and how to take the medication, and potential side effects. As use of these programs becomes increasingly widespread, the incidence of inappropriate medications and incorrect dosages will hopefully decline.

One Boston-area hospital recently installed a new computer system that tracks every detail of a patient's care, and presents a list of appropriate doses when a doctor orders a prescription. A surveillance program also scans the patient's medical record for incompatible medications. As new entries are made on the patient's chart, the computer searches for changes that might necessitate withdrawing the prescription. The computer is expected to eliminate 85 percent of ordering errors and 50 percent of all drug injuries.

WOMEN AS VICTIMS OF MALPRACTICE

Women bear more than their share of the medical malpractice risk. They are especially vulnerable to malpractice from unnecessary surgery, risky contraceptive procedures, misdiagnoses of cancer, problematic prenatal care and delivery, and incompetent plastic surgery. Each of these "female" medical procedures is discussed below.

The problem of unnecessary surgery is well documented in the medical literature. Though estimates vary, at least 15 percent of the estimated 35,000,000 operations performed each year are unnecessary.[4] Hysterectomies, dilation and curettage, and Caesarean sections[5] are prominently featured in almost every listing of superfluous operations.

These medical procedures, though all too common, are far from benign. They change women's lives. Hysterectomies, about 600,000 of which are performed each year,[6] increase a woman's risk of heart disease and osteoporosis, bring on premature menopause, and have been linked to sexual problems.

A discussion of when a hysterectomy or any other medical procedure is or is not appropriate is beyond the scope of this book (and the expertise of its author). Most public libraries, however, have a collection of accessible medical literature that can help every woman participate in decisions about recommended surgical procedures. (See pages 11-12 for more on conducting your own medical research.)

Central to many women's claims of malpractice is the contention that their providers failed to impart the information needed to make appropriate treatment decisions. Take, for example, tubal ligation, a form of contraception. Doctors tend to portray the procedure as risk-free and guaranteed effective. This rosy picture is not entirely accurate. When a woman consents to the procedure without full knowledge of the risks involved, and then falls victim to one of the known risks, she can sue for malpractice.

Patients should not rely on one doctor as their sole source of information about a proposed medical procedure. They should get a second opinion from another doctor or the medical reference section of their local library. A wealth of medical literature documents the potential complications from tubal ligation.

Doctors also have a less than sterling record of diagnosing in good time cancers that affect only women. In fact, more lawsuits are brought against doctors on behalf of breast cancer patients than for patients with any other disease.[7]

Many women suffering from cancer have sued for malpractice when their cancers were misdiagnosed or left undiagnosed. Breast, uterine, and cervical cancer are all deadly if not caught early and properly treated. Especially with breast cancer, relatively few malpractice claims charge the doctor with negligent or inappropriate care once the condition has been diagnosed.

Most breast cancer malpractice claims result from doctors who negligently rely on a negative or inconclusive mammogram to rule out cancer. Mammography is not a perfect science, and doctors should not place exclusive reliance on a single test result. Other causes of delayed diagnoses include failure to detect a lump or an erroneous assumption that a lump is benign. Doctors who fail to follow up on breast irregularities that have been detected with a positive mammogram or manual breast exam may face liability, as might those who neglect to question their patients about nipple discharge and soreness when taking a medical history.

Women who bring a malpractice action alleging the doctor's failure to make a timely diagnosis of a cancerous condition have a difficult road to travel. They must prove that they stood a good likelihood of being cured *if* their condition had been diagnosed earlier.

Where the delay in diagnosis is a matter of weeks or even a few months (less than six), the plaintiff will have a hard time finding an expert willing to predict that the outcome would have been different with an earlier diagnosis. Delays of over six months are more easily linked to a predictable change in outcome. Where a delay of any duration was the result of clear negligence—say a misread mammogram—the plaintiff will probably win her case, despite the problem of proving a causal link between the delay and the outcome.

Cervical cancer, like breast cancer, is also frequently misdiagnosed or undiagnosed. When correctly diagnosed, virtually every case of invasive cervical cancer is preventable.

With cervical cancer, the guilty party is often the laboratory that has lost or switched test results or misplaced or misidentified test samples. Cervical cancer is rarely detected without an accurate Papanicolaou (Pap) smear test. Medical literature reveals numerous incidents of laboratories that have been charged with negligently analyzing and reporting Pap results.[8]

A doctor who places undue trust in a single laboratory test result may also face liability. Doctors should be familiar with the risk of both false negatives and false positive test results. As a precautionary measure, they should test at two or three independent laboratories patients with normal Pap results who are experiencing abnormal symptoms.

When an abnormal Pap smear test is reported back to the gynecologist, the gynecologist becomes responsible for notifying the patient, prescribing additional diagnostic tests to confirm or rule out the presence of cancerous signs, and treating the condition. A doctor who does not take the appropriate measures after learning about a positive Pap smear may face legal liability for malpractice.

Obstetricians are renowned for being the subject of large numbers of malpractice claims. The obstetrician's status as the paradigm malpractice defendant is almost inevitable. Obstetricians have an exceptionally difficult job to perform, and, when they err, they often shatter their patients' treasured dreams of bearing healthy children.

Obstetricians collect a wealth of clinical data over the course of a pregnancy. They document the fetus's heart rate, the mother's blood, urine, and medical history, genetic screenings, and the results of clinical examinations. They must then analyze and assimilate all of this data so that high-risk patients are identified and treated appropriately.

Computer software is finally starting to make the obstetrician's job a little easier. These programs help obstetricians interpret and organize complex and voluminous amounts of data. An obstetrician inputs patient data; the computer identifies those patients who are at greatest risk of particular complications, recommends tests and treatments, and spits out a handout to be given to the patient describing the nature of her condition and treatment.

Cosmetic surgery, though not as exclusively the domain of women as breast cancer, cervical cancer, and pregnancy, does attract more female patients than male. Tummy tuck, nose job, and face-lift patients are filing malpractice claims in record numbers. Many of these malpractice claims charge the doctor with using an untrained anesthesiologist, attempting to oversee the anesthesia himself while performing the surgery, or failing to have emergency procedures in place when the anesthesia goes awry.

PICKING QUALITY PROVIDERS

Here's a quiz. You have finally decided to get that face-lift you've been pondering for years. How do you go about selecting a qualified plastic surgeon?

1. Look in the Yellow Pages of the telephone book under S for Surgeon.

2. Schedule consultations with several potential candidates. Select the surgeon who promises to make you look like Racquel Welch.

3. Get a reference from your friend who recently underwent a similar procedure and has unqualified raves for her surgeon.

Congratulations to those of you who selected #3. A personal recommendation is one of the best ways to start looking for a qualified plastic surgeon, or any other physician.

You are primarily responsible for picking qualified health care providers. Unless you recognize and accept this responsibility, you place yourself at heightened risk of becoming a victim of medical malpractice. There is much you can do to protect yourself from incompetent practitioners.

One of your best defenses is your mouth. Ask questions!

If you are selecting a specialist, ask prospective candidates about board certification. Doctors who graduate from medical school are legally allowed to practice in any specialty, with or without the proper training. The only way to know whether a doctor has in fact completed the proper advanced training is if that doctor has been certified by the appropriate medical specialty board.

One note about plastic surgeons. Not every surgeon who performs plastic surgery is board certified in plastic surgery. Some highly qualified plastic surgeons are only board certified in another discipline, such as dermatology or otolaryngology. Surgeons who are not board certified in plastic surgery should not be rejected out of hand. You will want to know, however, the extent of their experience in plastic surgery. How long has the doctor been performing the type of procedure you are considering undergoing? How many procedures of this type does the doctor perform each month? What type of training does the doctor have in performing this type of procedure? If you do not have total confidence in the physician's experience and training, find yourself another specialist.

Say you find a doctor who swears on a stack of Bibles that she is a board certified plastic surgeon, or any other type of specialist. How do you know she is telling the truth?

The American Board of Medical Specialties has a toll-free number that you can call to verify a doctor's credentials. The number, 1-800-776-2378 (776-CERT), can be dialed Mondays through Fridays from 9 A.M. to 6 P.M., eastern standard time. When you call, an operator will tell you whether the doctor is board certified, the field of board certification, and the year of certification.

Another resource for confirming board certification is *The Official American Board of Medical Specialties (ABMS) Directory of Board Certified Medical Specialists.* This directory should be available in your local public library.

The American Medical Association (AMA) also provides to the public information about the credentials of its members. The AMA can be reached by calling 312-464-5000.

You will also want to question any prospective provider about his or her professional affiliations. Does the doctor have "privileges" to practice medicine at the most prestigious medical centers and hospitals in the area? Practitioners who are affiliated with reputable teaching facilities are generally among the most qualified members of their profession.

During your initial consultation, engage the doctor in a dialogue. Is the doctor forthcoming with information, both good *and* bad, about the treatment, recovery, potential complications, and fees? Are you comfortable discussing your fears and concerns with the doctor? Do you see eye-to-eye on such controversial issues as the role of alternative medicine and holistic health care?

As a final check into the doctor's qualifications, call the state health department's Office of Professional Medical Conduct. Has the physician ever been found guilty of misconduct? A finding of misconduct means you should probably continue your search for a different provider. (State departments of health are listed in appendix 1.)

GETTING QUALITY CARE FROM AN HMO

What if you do not have total freedom to select a physician? Members of some HMOs are only covered for care they receive from the group's own network of providers, with only limited exceptions. If you are one of the 2.6 million Americans who belong to an HMO, you might be wondering how HMO membership affects the quality of your medical care.

An advisory panel to the National Cancer Institute recently issued a report that addressed, among other things, whether HMO patients who had been diagnosed with cancer were receiving the best possible care when treated within their plan. The authors of the report concluded that perhaps they were not. In the opinion of the panelists, every cancer patient should have "freedom to choose the most appropriate provider" because "the most effective treatment for a patient's problem may be available only from an individual or institutional provider outside the plan."[9]

A second study presented at the 1995 annual meeting of the American Heart Association found that heart attack victims had a higher survival rate when treated by cardiologists rather than general practitioners. Many managed care insurance plans require that patients be seen by a primary care doctor before being referred to a specialist, such as a cardiologist. Some plans even give primary care doctors financial incentives to keep specialist referrals to a minimum. According to the study, patients admitted directly to a cardiology hospital ward had a 15 percent lower risk of dying within a year of the attack than patients treated by a general practitioner.

The possibility that membership in an HMO might be linked to higher mortality rates or lower quality of life among cancer or cardiac patients has sent tremors through the health care reform movement. Managed care is the darling of health care reform. The most well-respected reformers see managed care as the key to bringing America's health care spending under control.

Many experts, however, reject the notion that patients who belong to HMOs sacrifice quality of care. They say there is simply not enough accurate data to make reliable comparisons between patients treated within, and those treated outside, HMOs.

Take, for example, a study that compared the mortality rates of patients treated at cancer centers with those treated within an HMO. The study found that cancer center patients outlived the HMO patients.[10] This finding, standing alone, is terrifying to the millions of Americans enrolled in HMOs. However, its findings should not be taken on face value.

One problem with the study is that it did not include any quality of life measurements. The cancer center patients might have lived longer, but at what cost? Did they enjoy their additional days, months, or years of life, or was that time characterized by pain and incapacity? Dr. John Wasson, an expert on health care delivery at Dartmouth College, has noted that "Managed care . . . may be setting limits in ways that make a lot more sense than giving endless chemotherapy."[11]

The study comparing mortality rates of HMO and non-HMO patients has also been criticized for looking only at the *treatment* of these two groups of patients. The study did not consider how these groups compare when it comes to the timely *diagnosis* of their cancerous condition.

The only case-by-case comparision of treatment results of patients in HMOs and those treated in traditional medical practices found similar results in both groups, at least with respect to patients treated for high blood pressure or adult diabetes. The type of insurance plan selected did not affect whether the patient's blood sugar or blood pressure was under control, or the patient's mortality rate, after seven years.[12]

A different study found that elderly Americans enrolled in HMOs were actually *more* likely to have their cancers detected earlier than patients who were treated by private doctors. The HMO enrollees had a superior track record of receiving routine screenings, such as mammograms, Pap smears, fecal blood tests, and annual checkups.[13]

HMO patients may have an edge over their non-HMO counterparts when it comes to early diagnosis of cancer, but then what happens? Does a cancer patient who is treated through her HMO, as opposed to a cancer center, compromise the quality of her medical care? This question is the subject of heated debate between HMO directors and experts in cancer care.

HMO administrators defend the quality of care they provide to their members by citing their willingness to approve members for treatment outside the plan if no network providers are competent to provide the needed care. Dr. Lee Newcomer, the medical director of the United HealthCare Corporation, is one such administrator. He once said, "Many of the services that a cancer center can provide can also be provided in town by a local oncologist. And if the local oncologist says, 'Hey, I can't do this,' almost every HMO will say, 'OK. Where's the best center?' "[14]

HMO directors also insist that they are more honest with their members about the limitations of experimental treatments than are doctors who work at cancer centers. Cancer centers rely to a greater extent than HMOs on treatments that show some potential for success but have not yet been fully tested and proven effective. Patients treated at cancer centers are often encouraged to enroll in research studies of new treatments. HMO administrators argue that patients sign up for experimental treatments in the hope of being cured when, in fact, the likelihood of a beneficial outcome is remote.

So what's the bottom line? Do you take your life in your hands when you enroll in an HMO? Are you better off paying for your care with traditional fee-for-service insurance that allows you to select your providers?

There is certainly evidence that cancer centers do provide the best care for cancer patients. These centers are more likely to have on-staff specialists with extensive experience treating each type of cancer. Also, these large centers are usually the first to employ new treatments that have been proven to be effective.

Do not, however, feel consigned to second-class medical care if you belong to an HMO. There are steps you can take to get the best possible care within your plan.

The place to start is with your HMO primary care physician. After you have been diagnosed with a condition that requires the services of a specialist, review the list of network specialists with your primary care physician. Request that he or she recommend you to the best-qualified specialist.

Ask the HMO for information about the recommended specialist's credentials.

Is the specialist affiliated with the most reputable medical centers? Where did he or she receive training? Some HMOs are more forthcoming with this information than others. Use the resources discussed earlier in this section to confirm board certification and uncover charges of misconduct.

At your first consultation with the specialist, make sure he or she is equipped to provide you with the best possible care. To make this determination, you must know something about the available treatments for your medical condition. You will be stymied in your efforts to evaluate the adequacy of the network provider if you do not know what constitutes the "best" care. To learn more about the care you need, you will have to do some medical research on your own.

Say, for instance, you have been diagnosed with cancer of the uterus, ovaries, or cervix. You have learned by researching success rates among cancer patients that patients with these three cancers fare best when treated by a gynecological oncologist. You look in your HMO's directory of specialists. No gynecological oncologist. You are not surprised, since most gynecological oncologists are affiliated with cancer centers.

You schedule a consultation with the most highly qualified specialist your HMO has to offer. Find out as much as you can about that specialist's training and experience. How does it differ from that of a gynecological oncologist? If you decide you still want to be treated by a gynecological oncologist, put your concerns and findings in a letter to the HMO requesting approval of treatment outside the plan with a gynecological oncologist. As long as you can prove a need for care that cannot be provided through a network practitioner, and are persistent, you should eventually get the coverage you are seeking.

Here's another example. You are diagnosed with colon cancer. An HMO surgeon recommends a colostomy. He proposes cutting an artificial opening for the discharge of waste.

You go to the library for a second opinion and learn that cancer specialists at the local teaching hospital have started using a combination of chemotherapy and radiation to treat your type of cancer. You also learn about an operation for colon cancer that does not entail a colostomy. The HMO surgeon you consult knows nothing about these alternative courses of treatment. You argue to the plan administrator that the treatment you need is not available within the HMO. Once again, if you're willing to fight the good fight, you should be covered for treatment outside the plan.

You should pursue your own medical research with an eye toward getting answers to the following questions: What is the current state of medical research into your ailment? What are the risks and benefits of alternative modes of treatment? Who has written articles that pertain most closely to your medical condition? With which medical institutions are these authors affiliated? Where are these institutions located? If your research reveals that you need a type of specialist or treatment that is not available within your HMO, insist on coverage outside your plan.

Medical research has never been easier for the layperson. Depending on your financial resources and computer savvy, you can conduct your research through a local library, your personal computer, or a paid research service. Each of these options is considered in turn.

Almost every public library has a collection of medical texts. Some large libraries also let you access medical information through computer searches. You type in the topic of interest, and the computer searches a database of medical information. A plethora of information quickly appears on the screen for your perusal. The librarian should be able to assist you in searching CD-ROM and MED-LINE databases.

If the resources of your local library are limited, you may have to take your search to a medical library. Contact your local medical society for a referral to a nearby medical library open to the public. You may even be able to use the medical society's own library. Patients receiving treatment in a hospital or medical center should ask whether the facility has an on-site library that is available for patient use.

Those of you with a personal computer and modem can conduct medical research from the comfort of home. You can start by signing up for an on-line computer service. These on-line services can be your ticket onto the Internet, the so-called information highway.

Once on the Internet, you will have immediate access to hundreds of medical databases. At your fingertips you will find a dazzling array of resource materials from a mind-boggling assortment of sources worldwide. You will also be able to communicate with medical professionals and other interested parties on electronic "bulletin boards." These bulletin boards allow on-line users to communicate electronically by posting messages on their computers. They can share information about the latest treatments, diagnostic techniques, and specialists, and discuss other topics of interest.

If you would like someone else to do your computer research for you, call one of the services listed below. These services find medical information for you. The Center for Medical Consumers in New York City has rated eight of these services. You can call the center at 212-674-7105 for ratings information.

➤ CANCERFAX   301-402-5874
    If you have a fax machine, you can fax in a request for free reports on specific cancers from the National Cancer Institute.

➤ THE HEALTH RESOURCE   501-329-5272
    For a fee ($295 for a cancer search and $195 for all other topics), you will receive at least 50 pages of information covering conventional treatments, international data, alternative treatments, and a list of specialists.

➤ H.E.R.M.E.S.   1-800-484-9863 (ext. 5773)
    For a fee of $49.50 you will get three sets of articles with some citations,

for $89.95 you will get 10 articles, and for $179.50 you will get 20 articles including, if available, a list of practitioners.

➤ SCHINE ON-LINE   1-800-FIND-CURE

For a fee ($189 for a cancer search and $110 for all other topics), you will receive largely technical information from medical and scientific journals covering treatment options, foreign studies, and clinical trials.

➤ PLANETREE   415-923-3681

For a fee of $20 to $35, you can receive a bibliography of indexed articles; the fee for the text of the articles is $100.

➤ MEDSCAN   1-800-MED-8145

For a fee that ranges from about $100 to $300, depending on the extensiveness of the search and the medical topic, Medscan will provide articles, citations, a glossary, and lists of specialists, resource organizations, holistic practitioners, and research projects.

Another good source of medical information is the Federal Agency for Health Care Policy and Research. The agency pays Patient Outcomes Research Teams across the country to identify the most effective treatments for a range of disorders. Although health care providers are not required to follow the Team's recommendations as to the most effective treatments, the recommendations are issued in the hope of standardizing medical treatment across the country. To get a copy of the free patient treatment guides, you can call the agency toll-free at 1-800-358-9295 and speak to a representative.

Health care reformers who praise managed care as the answer to America's health care crisis have promised not to achieve cost savings at the expense of quality of care. They have put forward proposals to monitor quality of care among competing HMOs.

The proposals envision publicizing information about the relative performance of every HMO. Health care consumers could then use this information to select providers who offer the highest quality care at the most reasonable prices. Market forces would drive out of business HMOs that provided inferior care.

There is, however, a hitch. Techniques for accurately measuring the quality of medical care remain elusive. Some experts estimate that we are still years away from developing reliable methods of gathering and analyzing health care data.

Today, the most widely accepted system for measuring the quality of medical providers is called outcomes analysis. Outcomes analysis uses treatment results to measure quality of care. Healthy patients are traced to competent providers. Warts and all, outcomes analysis is the best there is—at least for now.

The science of outcomes analysis is still in its infancy. The U.S. Health Care Financing Administration (HCFA) only started using outcomes analysis in the mid-1980s, when it issued yearly reports comparing the treatment of Medicare patients at 5,000 different hospitals across the country. The reports looked at the mortality rates at the targeted institutions. The rates were adjusted to account for the patient mix and risk factors. Facilities with mortality rates outside the predicted range became the subject of investigation.

Not surprisingly, hospitals that received the poorest ratings with outcomes analysis challenged the process. They argued that the analysis failed to give due credit to those facilities that treated the sickest patients, which were mostly public hospitals. In 1993 a new administrator assumed the helm at HCFA and nixed the hospital rankings.

Critics of outcomes analysis charge the process with yielding inaccurate and misleading results. Kenneth E. Raske, president of the Greater New York Hospital Association, a trade group, is one such critic. Mr. Raske sees outcomes analysis as a useful tool for medical professionals and health care reformers, but not for consumers. The results of outcomes analysis, according to Raske, cannot be understood without a certain degree of sophistication. When the studies are published in newspapers, the public misunderstands and misuses the findings.[15]

Dr. James S. Todd, senior deputy executive vice-president of the American Medical Association, agrees. As might be expected, Dr. Todd is especially critical of outcomes analysis of doctors. According to Dr. Todd, "There are many other things that influence outcomes such as the hospital, its ancillary services, associated diseases, and the patient himself . . . I don't think we will live long enough to see outcomes technology as a useful tool for the public."[16]

Despite its immaturity as a science, outcomes analysis is still the most popular method of evaluating quality of care. The Federal Agency for Health Care Policy and Research uses outcomes data to compare the effectiveness of different treatments and to issue uniform treatment guidelines. Some state governments use outcomes analysis to identify ineffective treatments and incompetent doctors and hospitals. In the private sector, insurance companies, business groups, and large employers use outcomes reports to select among competing health care networks.

If consumer groups have anything to say about it, outcomes analysis is here to stay. Public and private health care consumers want access to data about their prospective providers' treatment success rates. A 1995 study by Louis Harris and Associates found that 66 percent of those surveyed would like to see report cards for hospitals, 58 percent would like to see ratings of physicians, and 52 percent would like ratings for health plans.[17]

The Center for Medical Consumers, a health advocacy group in New York City, dismisses the medical industry's professed concern about confusing the public as nothing more than propaganda from providers who resent monitoring by outcomes analysts. Perhaps the director of the center, Arthur Levin, said it best: "Medicine has always claimed it is a science until you ask for data. Then, it is an art."[18]

New York and Pennsylvania are the two states to make the greatest use of outcomes analysis. Pennsylvania has been rating hospitals on cost and quality for a total of fifty-seven treatments since 1988. New York State began ranking hospitals based on deaths from coronary artery bypass graft surgeries in 1990; in 1991, it began publicizing information about specific surgeons.[19]

Interestingly, despite the distribution of 10,000 reports documenting the relative death rate from bypass surgery at Pennsylvania hospitals, the medical center rated as one of the least expensive and highest-quality facilities for bypass procedures has seen no increase in patients after publication of the state's findings.[20]

An article in *The New England Journal of Medicine* that was critical of New York's method of ranking hospitals and cardiac surgeons exposes some of the difficulties inherent in outcomes analysis. Surgeons' ranks often fluctuate greatly from year to year. In one year, 46 percent of surgeons moved from one half of the list to the other. This fickleness led the authors to question the reliability of the ranking. Also, New York counts only deaths that occur in hospitals. The authors noted that the ranking might underestimate the death rates of patients who were treated in hospitals that discharge their patients to their homes after treatment options have been exhausted.[21] There is also concern that New York doctors refer their high-risk patients out of state, and exaggerate the risk of their cardiac patients.[22]

Outcomes analysis of who is doing which procedures has yielded some surprising, and disturbing, results. Low-volume hospitals perform half of all Medicare angioplasties, despite compelling evidence that hospitals and doctors who perform large numbers of angioplasty procedures have a lower mortality rate than do low-volume providers. The likelihood that a woman will have a hysterectomy ranges from 20 to 70 percent, depending on where she lives. The likelihood that a man with an enlarged prostrate will undergo surgery ranges from 15 percent to 60 percent, also depending on where he lives. According to these numbers, a lot of us are either getting surgery we don't need or are not getting surgery we do need.

Another source of information that is available to you when selecting a medical provider—whether you are looking for a hospital, home care agency, long-term care institution, or mental health care organization—is the Joint Commission on Accreditation of Healthcare Organizations (JCAHO). The JCAHO evaluates and accredits more than 11,000 health care organizations nationwide. Accredited facilities are required to maintain certain standards of care or risk losing accreditation. The JCAHO makes available to the public for a $30 fee a Hospital Performance Report. To get information on ordering the report, call the JCAHO at 708-916-5600. In addition to the report itself, you will get informational brochures on how to select quality health care organizations.

There are also ratings available for HMOs. Unlike other rating systems, however, the HMO-rating system is of singularly little benefit to consumers.

The problems with the HMO rating system are manifold. For starters, HMOs usually rate themselves. Their self-ratings are not based on uniform data sources, and the integrity of their studies are not verified by independent sources.

To make matters worse, most HMOs rate themselves on patient satisfaction rather than on quality of care. They pay more attention to short waits for doctors and open phone lines than to treatment outcomes. They highlight the percentage of patients who receive preventive care without considering mortality rates among their members.

Most HMOs engage in self-rating as a promotional measure to attract new enrollees. They use the ratings to portray themselves in the best possible light.

Many state health departments and insurance departments maintain records of complaints filed against HMOs. Some rank HMOs by the number of complaints received. These rankings are usually available to the public upon request. (State departments of health and insurance are listed in appendices 1 and 3 respectively.)

New York legislators recently proposed a Health Care Bill of Rights that would regulate quality of care among HMOs. The legislation would require HMOs to offer an adequate choice of competent providers, limit out-of-pocket expenses, implement internal grievance procedures, and provide members with detailed information about the plan's features and limitations. Restrictions on tests, treatment options, referrals, and services would have to be disclosed, as would the number of claims denied, and results of consumer appeals. To date, no state has passed such legislation.

POLICING THE MEDICAL PROFESSION

The public's most potent line of defense against incompetent medical practitioners is the state licensing board. (A state-by-state listing of licensing boards appears in appendix 4.) The state licensing board authorizes physicians and other health care professionals to practice medicine within the state's borders. Only a licensing board has the power to suspend or revoke a medical license.

As part of their duties, licensing boards are supposed to make sure that practitioners who provide substandard care are not allowed to practice medicine in the state. Unfortunately, not every licensing board has the same understanding of what constitutes a "bad" doctor. Furthermore, licensing boards are not uniform in their perception of their mission. Some boards believe that their job is to discipline doctors, while others attempt to rehabilitate physicians who provide substandard care.

Consumer groups generally like to see state boards take disciplinary measures against physicians who are found to have rendered negligent care to their patients. The Public Citizen Health Research Group, for example, advocates that boards suspend and revoke the licenses of doctors who are found guilty of malpractice. Boards should strip doctors of the privilege of practicing medicine, the group argues, when the doctors breach the public's trust by providing substandard care.

This approach does not always work, especially in rural areas where boards cannot be so cavalier about ousting deficient practitioners. Sometimes the doctor who has been found to have provided negligent care is the only game in town. Is a doctor who occasionally provides substandard care better than no doctor at all?

Where a board is presented with a situation where suspending or terminating the doctor's license could leave residents at greater risk of harm, the board may attempt rehabilitation. The doctor may be required to undergo additional training, start counseling, take a competency examination, and/or submit to ongoing monitoring as a condition of retaining his or her license.

There are risks associated with both the rehabilitative and disciplinary approaches to medical misconduct.

Boards that respond to medical wrongdoing with exacting punishment are in danger of alienating the medical community. Most state boards rely on other health care professionals to report instances of incompetency and impairment among their colleagues.

Often practitioners report their coworkers to state boards in the hope of securing help for their troubled colleagues in the profession. Doctors may be less inclined to report their associates to a board whose response is purely punitive. Boards that lose the cooperation of other practitioners are at a distinct disadvantage when it comes to identifying and remedying medical incompetency.

Boards that attempt to rehabilitate troubled health care providers might encourage doctors to self-police their profession, but these boards face a different risk: A problem that gives rise to an initial complaint may be allowed to recur.

Take the situation of a doctor who injures a patient while under the influence of alcohol. The board intervenes and requires the doctor to attend Alcoholics Anonymous meetings. The doctor, unable to control his drinking, suffers a relapse. While inebriated, he injures another patient. The board is roundly criticized for failing to take strong enough action against the practitioner.

Depending on state law, board actions may or may not be a matter of public record. A state law may, for example, require boards to publish all disciplinary actions except where the physician's problem relates to a medical condition, such as a physical or mental impairment, chemical dependency, or AIDS. Other states may keep confidential the identities of practitioners who have been the subject of board action.

There are compelling arguments both for and against public disclosure. The argument favoring disclosure is obvious: The public has a right to know if the physicians treating them have ever committed acts of malpractice. Arguments against disclosure are premised on public policy considerations. Society spends billions of dollars to educate its doctors. Federal tax dollars are used to fund medical school research programs, and hospital patients pay the salaries of new doctors who are completing their medical education with practical experience. The disclosure of a board action can bring to a grinding halt the career of a doctor who is the subject of the proceeding. When that occurs, society loses the benefit of its investment.

Public disclosure of board actions also risks discouraging troubled practitioners from reporting themselves to state boards. As long as the proceedings are kept private, doctors in crisis can get help putting their lives back on track without committing professional suicide.

State boards do not have an enviable job. They must find bad doctors, prove medical wrongdoing, issue sanctions, and defend their sanctions in court . . . all on a shoestring budget. Impediments to the effectiveness of state boards are discussed below.

PROBLEMS FACING STATE BOARDS

Boards learn about bad doctors from primarily two sources—dissatisfied patients and other doctors. In about forty states, medical professionals are legally obligated to report to the licensing board their colleagues' suspicious behavior. The efficacy of a state's reporting laws seems to depend, at least in part, on whether the complainant's identity is revealed. In the majority of states, the board becomes the named accuser if a preliminary investigation reveals evidence of wrongdoing. The identity of the initial complainant remains confidential. This seems to work quite well. In those states where the complainant can be identified during the discovery process that precedes the board hearing, fewer doctors report the misdeeds of their colleagues.

Some state reporting laws exempt individual physicians. Hospitals, malpractice insurers, medical associations, the state's attorney general, and other state agencies must report medical wrongdoing to the state licensing board, but doctors are not required to expose unfit colleagues. The exemption of individual physicians is difficult to understand. A doctor who witnesses and reports another doctor's wrongdoing can nip the problem in the bud. Hospitals and other entities usually learn about a physician's ineptitude only after a pattern of negligence has emerged—a costly delay.

A federal reporting law requires hospitals to report disciplinary actions to the state licensing board. There is some evidence that hospitals do not deserve to be entrusted with this duty of exposing medical incompetency.

Hospitals have traditionally been reluctant to get involved in extended state board actions that could culminate in the suspension or revocation of a doctor's medical license. Take, for example, a well-respected hospital in Salt Lake City. A hospital spokesman acknowledged to a reporter that the facility has the capability to track the best and worst surgeons with an advanced computer system, yet conceded that the hospital does not report "bad apples" to the state licensing board because "you have to construct a 'safe' environment where doctors trust you. Any time you start taking names, you're going to start a cycle of fear . . ."[23] An unstated reason some hospitals are reluctant to report the negligence of staff physicians to state boards is the fear of being sued by the chastised doctor.

Hospitals that are subject to reporting laws have been known to circumvent their legal obligations. They want bad doctors off their staff, but they are unwilling to take the extra step of reporting the doctor to the state board. They may ask the physician to resign, take a temporary leave, get into a drug or alcohol treatment program, or attend continuing education classes in exchange for the hospital's silence. Aware of these strategies, some state boards investigate the circumstances surrounding every permanent and temporary hospital staff resignation to confirm the voluntary nature of the physician's departure.

In March 1995 the federal inspector general reported that between September 1, 1990, and December 31, 1993, three-quarters of American hospitals reported disciplining no physicians. Seventy-six percent of all hospitals reported no suspensions of more than thirty days. Federal health officials immediately expressed skepticism that so few doctors are botching patient care.[24]

State boards do not always depend on outside sources to identify unfit practitioners. Some boards track down medical malpractice on their own by surveying pharmacists, reviewing medical records, and conducting on-site inspections.

You may think all "bad" doctors are the same, but there are actually two types of "bad" doctors. There are impaired doctors, who provide substandard care as a result of drug or alcohol abuse or a psychiatric or psychological illness, and there are incompetent doctors, who lack the skill or training to provide effective medical care.

Generally, impaired doctors are easier to identify and treat or discipline than incompetent doctors. Many impaired doctors reveal themselves to licensing boards; few incompetent doctors turn themselves in. Colleagues of impaired doctors frequently report their coworkers to boards; medical professionals are reluctant to report coworkers' incompetence.

In addition, the impairment standard is easier to apply than the incompetency standard. A doctor who treats a patient while under the influence of drug or alcohol is impaired and clearly should not be practicing medicine. End of story. A family doctor who misses a tiny tumor when viewing a patient's X-ray scan may or may not be negligent, depending on the standard of care to which he is held.

There are more impaired doctors practicing medicine than anyone wants to know. The percentage of doctors who are alcoholic hovers between 10 and 15 percent, and between 15 and 20 percent have some form of mental illness. These percentages mirror the figures of the general population. Doctors fare worse, however, when it comes to drug abuse. As many as 10 percent of doctors abuse drugs, while this problem afflicts only about 2 percent of the general population.

State boards enjoy greater success disciplining impaired doctors than they do in disciplining incompetent doctors. According to the Public Citizen Health Research Group's 1991 edition of "9,479 Questionable Doctors," less than 10 percent of state-board actions were taken against doctors who provided substandard or negligent care.

Many state licensing boards are limited by a scarcity of resources in their ability to take action against incompetent doctors who provide substandard care.

The boards lack the time, money, manpower, and experience needed to ferret these doctors out.

The process that follows the identification of a potentially unfit provider can take several years and cost many thousands of dollars to complete. Herein lies the rub. State boards can afford neither the time nor the money needed to be a truly effective mechanism for policing the medical profession.

Many state boards are strapped for funds. Although the boards generate revenue by collecting licensure fees from in-state professionals, these fees often pass into the general state treasury. The state legislatures then allocate back to the boards a minimum portion of the funds. State boards across the country perpetually fight for the right to fund themselves with their own licensure fees.

Many licensed health care professionals exploit their state board's budgetary constraints. They do not cooperate with ongoing investigations, knowing that the board is understaffed and overworked. They are familiar with the huge backlog of cases waiting to be investigated. They may have heard that the board's staff is inexperienced and undertrained.

Boards frequently put their investigatory dollars into the cases that are easiest to win in court. Their reasoning is sound. They cannot afford to take every case to trial. They cannot afford to lose the cases they do decide to litigate. If they repeatedly lose in court, doctors will not take the threat of being taken to a board hearing seriously. The boards must win in court.

The cases that boards are most likely to pursue into litigation are those that can be successfully prosecuted with a minimum investment of time and money. Board actions that duplicate sanctions already imposed by a neighboring state are among the cheapest and easiest to prosecute and win. A doctor who loses his license in State X comes to State Y to practice medicine. The State Y licensing board begins a proceeding to prevent him from practicing medicine in that state as well. Not surprisingly, these types of actions represent the largest number of state board actions.

As already mentioned, malpractice cases grounded in claims of negligence are among the most difficult to prove. They often take a considerable investment of time and money. The board must overcome an onerous burden of proof—which varies from state to state—to win its case against the doctor.

The most common burden of proof in board actions is "clear and convincing evidence." The best way to illustrate the burden of this standard is to compare it with the standard that applies in most civil malpractice tort suits—a "preponderance of the evidence."

A patient suing for malpractice in a civil suit proves the doctor's negligence by having more evidence of wrongdoing than the defendant has in his defense. As long as the plaintiff can prove that *it is more likely than not* that the defendant rendered substandard care, the plaintiff will prevail. Boards that require clear and convincing evidence of wrongdoing will not penalize a doctor based on a mere preponderance of the evidence. They need more proof.

As if state boards didn't have enough problems, between their tight budgets and exacting burden of proof, they must fight like the dickens to get bad doctors to stop practicing medicine. The typical doctor who loses a board hearing will file an appeal. Doctors invest too much time and money in their medical careers to lose their license without a fight.

The appeal process is tortuously slow and costly, not to mention unfair. The board is the proverbial David fighting the infinitely better armed Goliath. The doctor often has experienced legal minds on his side; the board may be defended by second- and third-year lawyers. The doctor and his insurer can afford to fly in medical experts from across the country; the board may depend on a panel of volunteer medical experts.

While the appeal is pending, many courts "stay" the action of the state board. An action that is stayed does not go into effect. The doctor who is the subject of the state board sanction is allowed to continue practicing medicine. Courts often grant the stay out of fear of wrongfully revoking the doctor's license, causing the doctor irreparable harm, and then being overturned on appeal. Unless there is compelling proof that the doctor is an imminent threat to the public, the doctor's interest in protecting his medical license will often prevail over the public's interests in being protected against potentially unfit physicians.

In a typical case, a doctor being investigated by a board can continue practicing medicine through two years of investigation and board hearings and five years of appeals. Finally, after seven years have passed and tens of thousands of dollars in legal fees have been expended, the courts usually implement the board's sanction. Appellate courts rarely overturn medical board decisions.

Some states will summarily suspend the doctor who is the subject of the proceeding without waiting for the full appeal process to run its course, but only in cases where the doctor poses a clear and imminent threat to the public. Although so-called summary suspensions offer the benefit of stopping inept internists and other physicians from practicing medicine, their use is limited as a practical matter. Only doctors who are severely impaired or clearly dangerous to the public are usually the subject of summary suspensions. Negligent and incompetent doctors do not have much to fear from summary proceedings.

Dr. David Benjamin, the New York physician who was eventually convicted of murder in 1995 for botching a 1993 abortion, had first been reported in 1990. Although the state board found the charges sufficiently troublesome to merit a full hearing, it found that the doctor was not an "imminent danger" to the public because the charges were years old. It did not summarily suspend his license. During the appeal process, Dr. Benjamin botched the abortion that led to his conviction.

State licensing boards, though noble in their intentions, are subject to financial and political restrictions that hinder their ability to protect the public from unqualified licensed health care professionals. In 1994, less than one percent of U.S. physicians had their licenses revoked or suspended, or were formally reprimanded by a board for misconduct.[25]

If state boards are not protecting us against medical incompetence, who or what is doing the job?

There is an assortment of organizations, each of which assumes some aspect of physician oversight. There is the Drug Enforcement Administration (DEA), which is on the lookout for suspicious practices involving prescription drugs and controlled substances. There are malpractice insurance companies, who encourage their insureds to provide quality care. There are Peer Review Organizations (PROs), which are physicians under contract with federal and state governments, that are supposed to maintain high standards of care among Medicare-certified (and sometimes Medicaid-certified and private) providers. Finally, there is self-policing within the medical profession through informal colleague and partnership review systems and impaired-physician rehabilitation programs. This collection of doctor-watchers joins state licensing boards, at least in theory, to ensure the competency of our medical providers.

Patchwork, ineffective, haphazard, uncoordinated, inconsistent, and *disorganized* are just some of the adjectives that have been used to describe the existing system of health care quality control. Critics charge the DEA with failing to maintain adequate records of disciplinary actions that are taken against physicians' DEA certificates. They accuse PROs of being more concerned with saving money than with detecting unfit providers. Impaired-physician rehabilitation programs are found to be in too short supply to be truly effective.

One of the biggest problems with this disjointed approach to medical monitoring is the lack of effective communication. Unless channels of communication are open and flowing, one medical monitor does not know what the others are doing. The result is fatal inefficiency.

To some extent, the communication problem has been addressed by the National Practitioner's Data Bank (NPDB). The NPDB was established to facilitate communication for the purpose of coordinating the efforts of the variety of medical policing organizations. The NPDB, which is operated by the federal Health and Human Services' Division of Quality Assurances, went on-line on September 1, 1990. Since that date, every action taken by a state licensing board, hospital privilege board, the DEA, professional society, or malpractice insurer is listed in the NPDB.

The names of licensed health care professionals who make malpractice payments to patients are listed in the data bank, regardless of the size of the payment and regardless of whether the payment is made in settlement of a dispute or after verdict. Each and every malpractice payment is listed in the data bank.

Whenever a doctor applies to a hospital for employment or clinical privileges, the hospital is supposed to run the applicant's name through the data bank. Hospitals are also required to check the doctor's data bank report every two years after commencement of employment. Managed care plans, professional membership societies, state licensing boards, and other public and private entities may, but are not required to, also solicit information from the NPDB.

As of today, the NPDB is not open to the public. Although many consumer organizations advocate publicizing the identities of doctors who have been listed in the NPDB, Congress has thus far been unreceptive to such proposals.

Consumer groups have another complaint as well. They charge the data bank with not accurately portraying each physician's malpractice history, thanks to the "corporate shield" rule.

Injured patients who belong to managed care plans, such as HMOs, typically list the medical plan as the defendant instead of the allegedly incompetent physician. The corporate shield protects the doctor from liability by shifting responsibility for on-the-job wrongdoing to the doctor's employer. The physician's own identity often remains a secret. Congress has debated removing the so-called corporate shield in medical malpractice cases, but it has not yet done so.

Advocates of non-litigation approaches to resolving malpractice disputes, including arbitration, mediation, and other methods of alternative dispute resolution (ADR), also oppose the data bank, which they find to work at cross purposes. They charge the NPDB with discouraging compromise and settlement—the hallmarks of ADR.

These advocates say that the identities of doctors who are willing to settle their malpractice disputes should remain confidential. Doctors will be less inclined to offer disgruntled plaintiffs even a nominal sum of money to withdraw their charges if the doctor's reputation will be sullied anyway by an NPDB listing. Any doctor who is going to risk his professional reputation with an NPDB listing might as well take his chances with a jury. At least the jury might clear his name.

The government has conceded the merit of this concern. Federal health officials have considered changing the NPDB so that only malpractice payments that exceed a certain threshold amount are listed.

The American Medical Association (AMA) supports proposals that limit the reporting requirements of the NPDB. The AMA says the existing system unjustifiably tarnishes the names of practitioners who settle weak cases to avoid the hassle and expense of litigation, even if there is no proof of wrongdoing.

The AMA, among others, champions a $30,000 reporting threshold. They contend that doctors will pay up to $30,000 to dispose of cases where medical liability cannot be proved just to avoid the massive outlays of time, money, and emotional energy that it takes to defend a malpractice action. Thirty-thousand dollars is the so-called nuisance value of a bad malpractice case because even the weakest case cannot be defended for less than that sum of money. Cases that are settled for less than $30,000 are insignificant and do not warrant reporting.

Different groups have come up with different threshold amounts. The American Hospital Association and Physician Insurers Association of America have advocated a $50,000 threshold. Other trade groups have recommended specialty-based thresholds. With specialty-based thresholds, the threshold amount would depend on the accused's area of medical practice. For neurosurgeons, obstetricians, and other high-risk practitioners, the threshold has been targeted at $75,000 or $100,000. For family physicians the threshold would be lower, perhaps $30,000 or $50,000. Dentists would be held to an even lower threshold of $20,000 or

$30,000. Some reform proposals would apply different thresholds to different areas of the country.

As of today, claims need not exceed any threshold amount to qualify for inclusion in the data bank. Despite the urging of the AMA, the Secretary of the federal Health and Human Services has thus far rejected setting reporting thresholds. Although setting thresholds below which claims would not have to be reported to the data bank would probably save the government money by reducing the number of malpractice reports filed, there are other overriding concerns.

The most compelling argument against reporting thresholds is that they could corrupt the malpractice system by encouraging defendants to manipulate damage payments. If damage payments under $30,000 did not have to be reported, for example, plaintiffs could count on seeing record numbers of $29,999 offers of settlement. Defendant doctors would have every reason to offer settlements just below the threshold amount. Between 1983 and 1990, New Jersey experimented with a $25,000 reporting threshold. A government study found many doctors settling malpractice claims for $24,999 during this period of time. BIG SURPRISE!

Another danger associated with reporting thresholds is that practitioners could avoid a data bank listing by sharing liability with other providers. Large payments could be divided among multiple providers so that no single provider paid more than the threshold amount. Shared liability would satisfy the plaintiff's interest in maximizing his award of damages, and would keep all potential defendants out of the bank.

On the other side of the fence of those who advocate reporting thresholds are those who favor *expanding* the NPDB reporting requirements. Reporting malpractice *payments*, they argue, is not enough. Every malpractice *claim*, not just payment, should be listed in the data bank.

Malpractice claims should be listed, the argument goes, because they are of interest to patients even if they are not proof of malpractice. Listing claims is also more timely than listing payments. Years can pass before a malpractice claim culminates in a post-settlement or post-verdict payment. During the intervening years, patients remain in the dark about their practitioners' malpractice history.

If the NPDB is not the solution to the problem of monitoring the medical profession, perhaps the answer lies with periodic retesting of licensed physicians. Some consumer groups think medical licenses should come with an expiration date. Under this system, doctors who neglected to submit their medical records for audit and failed to pass a competency exam would not be granted a license renewal.

No state currently has a retesting law. New York is the only state that has even debated such legislation. Only a handful of boards that certify medical specialists have mandatory recertification programs.

Opponents of retesting cite cost as a major concern. They see the money that would have to be invested in the administration and enforcement of a retesting program as better spent on doctors who have already been identified as potential problems. Why waste money on doctors who appear to be providing quality care?

Selective testing has enjoyed a somewhat warmer reception. The goal of selective testing is to identify and document particular areas of medical weakness. The Federation of State Medical Boards has developed a Special Purpose Examination (or SPEX) that some boards use to question doctors who are the subject of a pattern of similar complaints. An accused doctor who fails the SPEX may automatically lose his or her license to practice medicine, at least for a period of time.

A final note about policing the medical profession. In recent years, state governments across the country have started to take a new approach toward disciplining doctors—criminal prosecution. Physicians who are responsible for wrongfully causing a patient's death have been indicted for murder.

In New York, Dr. David Benjamin was convicted of murder and sentenced to twenty-five years to life in prison when his patient bled to death following a botched abortion. Another New York practitioner, Dr. Gerald Einaugler, was sentenced to Riker's Island when he was convicted of two misdemeanor charges in connection with the death of a nursing home patient. In Denver, an anesthesiologist was charged with manslaughter when he fell asleep during routine ear surgery and an eight-year-old died as a result.

In the opinion of Dr. Wolfe of the Public Citizen's Health Research Group, the medical profession has no one but itself to blame for forcing the public's hand. If doctors had been more responsible about policing themselves, resort to criminal sanctions would never have become necessary.[26]

The American Medical Association disagrees. The threat of malpractice and civil sanctions are punishment enough if a doctor negligently causes a patient's death. Doctors should not be sent to jail for making a mistake, no matter how egregious the error might have been. Doctors are, after all, only human.

BRINGING A MALPRACTICE LAWSUIT

You might be surprised to learn that only one out of eight or ten patients who is injured as a result of a provider's negligence decides to sue. You might be even more surprised to learn *why* they decide to sue. Research shows the decision often has nothing to do with money.

A study was conducted of patients and relatives who had commenced legal malpractice proceedings against a medical provider.[27] Interestingly, a breakdown in doctor-patient communication seemed to be a greater predictor of the likelihood of suit than the severity of the resulting injury. Patients were most likely to sue when their doctors failed to provide a clear explanation of how and why the treatment error occurred. Also, patients were less forgiving, and more inclined to litigate, when their doctors refused to apologize for what had occurred.

The researchers concluded that there are four motivating forces that lead injured patients to sue their doctors. First, plaintiffs want explanations. They want defendants to completely and satisfactorily disclose all of the whys and wherefores of the adverse event. Second, plaintiffs want accountability. They want defendants to confront the damage they caused and pay (not only monetarily) for their negligence. Third, plaintiffs want to protect others. They want to promote high standards of medical care so that the same problem does not recur. And fourth, plaintiffs want compensation. They want to be covered for their actual monetary losses, their pain and suffering, and their anticipated future medical and care-related expenses.

In terms of compensation, the typical malpractice plaintiff seeks two types of damages; compensation for economic losses and compensation for non-economic losses. Economic losses include the injured patient's past and future medical expenses and lost income. Non-economic losses include pain and suffering, loss of companionship, and loss of quality of life.

There is nothing very interesting about economic damages. They are generally relatively easy to quantify.

Suppose, for example, that the injured patient was a 50-year-old bank executive who was earning $50,000 a year before he suffered brain damage as a result of a surgeon's negligence. He could not return to his prior position with the bank and faced the prospect of permanent unemployment. He already had $20,000 in outstanding medical bills, and his expenses were mounting. Daily physical therapy sessions were only partly covered by insurance, as was his psychiatric treatment for depression. In addition, he had to have his home modified to accommodate his wheelchair, and he was installing a whirlpool bath for therapeutic purposes.

His total economic loss is based on his future earning potential (fifteen or twenty more years of work with standard raises and bonuses), past ($20,000) and future (ongoing physical and psychiatric therapy) medical expenses, and other disability-related expenses (such as home modifications). Although counsel for the plaintiff and defendant may dispute the need for a private whirlpool bath, or the plaintiff's projected earning capacity, that's about it. The two sides are rarely very far apart in their estimation of the plaintiff's economic losses.

When it comes to assessing non-economic losses, on the other hand, the lawyers take off their gloves. The largest component of most awards for non-economic damages is usually compensation for the injured patient's pain and suffering. Given the difficulties inherent in quantifying pain and suffering, the subject is ripe for lawyerly wrangling.

Pain and suffering includes both physical and psychological pain. Emotional distress, mental anguish, loss of companionship (or "consortium" in legal lingo), and loss of the ability to enjoy life's pleasures ("hedonic damages") all figure into the valuation of pain and suffering.

The million dollar damages often sought for pain and suffering are arbitrary. When the parents of a fifteen-year-old patient with a botched nose job sue the surgeon for $1 million to compensate their daughter for the humiliation she will feel every day for the rest of her life when she goes out in public, they are picking a number out of their hat. The actual amount of damages available to them will depend on the trends of jury verdicts in their region of the country.

Similarly, when a thirty-year-old housewife and mother of two young sons dies on the operating table after the anesthesiologist accidentally administers the incorrect dosage of anesthesia, the husband can sue the anesthesiologist for $2 million compensation for lost support and companionship and another $2 million compensation for his children, who must grow up without their mother's loving guidance. The husband's actual recovery will reflect the local jury's sympathies for his family's unfortunate predicament and its attitude toward the medical profession.

Often the plaintiff in a malpractice action recovers both economic and non-economic damages. Return, for a moment, to the example of the thirty-year-old housewife. In addition to the non-economic damages, the husband may also be entitled to economic damages based on the cost of hiring someone to do the household cooking, cleaning, and laundry and care for the children. In the typical malpractice case, the award for non-economic damages is larger than the award for economic damages.

The three sweetest words you can whisper into the ear of a malpractice attorney are *pain and suffering*. The pain and suffering component of a malpractice award is the wild card. Anything can happen. Juries can, and have, awarded multimillion dollar pain and suffering awards to injured patients and their families.

The goal of plaintiffs' lawyers is clear: Win the jury's sympathy. Sympathetic juries are most inclined to make generous awards for pain and suffering.

One way lawyers who represent malpractice plaintiffs appeal to the sympathy of the jury is to put the injured patient on the stand. The lawyers ask their clients to describe their physical pain as graphically as possible for the jury. The lawyers may suggest highly descriptive adjectives, such as *excruciating, agonizing,* or *piercing* to describe the pain. They may encourage their clients to use illustrative analogies, such as the pain of a dentist's drill hitting a nerve. They may ask their clients to recall their greatest pleasures in life—work? sports? gardening? playing with the kids?—and describe how life has changed now that these activities are no longer feasible.

Occasionally plaintiff's counsel will call to the stand expert witnesses to help value damages. Medical experts testify about pain and incapacity, psychological experts discuss the nature of sorrow and grief, and forensic experts use quasi-scientific models to quantify pain and suffering. Since there is no real "science" to computing non-economic damages, the testimony of forensic experts is especially vulnerable to being attacked on cross-examination as arbitrary and unsubstantiated.

Expert witnesses are especially poorly suited to quantify "diminished quality of life" (or "hedonic") damages. These damages are intended to compensate the injured party for the lost ability to delight in life's pleasures.

Despite the shortcomings of expert testimony when it comes to valuing a plaintiff's inability to enjoy a pain-free stroll on a moonlit beach, lawyers do not give up. They use all the tools in their litigation arsenal to quantify the unquantifiable. They call to the stand forensic economists to apply "value of life" scales, and implore the jury to imagine life without such joys as riding a bicycle, reading a book, or going to the theater. Occasionally courts disallow testimony regarding the value of hedonic damages on the grounds that such testimony lacks scientific foundation.

Courts may dismiss a claim for hedonic damages when there is evidence that the plaintiff is not fully aware of his or her inability to enjoy life's pleasures. The injured party must be able to appreciate his or her restrictions in order for the damages to be compensable. Many state courts do not even allow separate awards for so-called hedonic damages.

How much emotional distress is enough emotional distress to support a claim for non-economic damages? This determination is, to a large extent, left to the discretion of the courts, as the following two examples demonstrate.

In one case, the parents of a baby who died days after birth as a result of a doctor's malpractice sued to recover damages. On appeal, the court found that the parents had failed to prove that their emotional distress caused physical problems, destroyed their basic emotional security, or significantly interfered with their professional or social lives. The court concluded: "The worry and stress that attend the birth of every child will not suffice, nor will upset which every parent feels when something goes wrong in the delivery room [to support a claim for damages for emotional distress]."

In another case, a mother sued for damages when a doctor's negligence left her year-old son permanently deaf. In that case, the appellate court was far more sympathetic. The court upheld the mother's award for pain and suffering out of respect for "the society, companionship, comfort, love, and solace" that exists between parent and child.

In the past, loss of companionship claims were available only to surviving spouses and mothers of injured infants. This has changed over time. Now growing numbers of state courts are allowing children, parents, siblings, and grandparents to recover damages for loss of companionship as long as the claimant has suffered psychologically—by losing out on the pleasure of watching a healthy grandchild mature, playing catch with a brother, or hearing a parent's words of advice. A client who has also suffered physical harm, perhaps insomnia or a gastric disorder, has an even stronger claim for damages.

In a malpractice action, the size of the damage award usually determines the size of the attorney's fee. Most malpractice attorneys charge a contingency fee. If the plaintiff loses, the attorney gets nothing. If the plaintiff wins, the attorney typically gets one-third of the award. Some states have adopted a sliding fee scale so the percentage of the award payable to the attorney drops as the size of the award increases.

Where the projected award is below $250,000, the would-be plaintiff might have trouble finding a malpractice attorney willing to take the case. Malpractice litigation is very costly and time-consuming, and most attorneys look for a sizable payoff at the end.

The magnitude of awards for non-economic damages is, in large part, responsible for the push to reform the legal malpractice system. Lawyers for doctors and hospitals argue that as long as the system allows plaintiffs to recover inflated sums of money as alleged compensation for unprovable pain and suffering, medical providers will continue to pay onerous malpractice insurance premiums and pass the costs along to health care consumers.

There is evidence that belies the widely held perception of jury awards as more a reflection of jurors' sympathy for plaintiffs and their hostility to doctors than a function of their effort to compensate plaintiffs for proven injuries. A 1993 study published in the *Annals of Internal Medicine,* for example, found that jury awards generally reflected the severity of the plaintiff's injuries, and that unjustified payments appeared to be uncommon.

Lawyers for plaintiffs have a question for critics of the existing malpractice system. Would you accept an offer of $1 million in exchange for a life of constant pain or the loss of a limb? Of course not. There is no adequate compensation when it comes to many types of medical malpractice. With the existing system, at least the jury can send a message to the medical profession that ineptitude will not be tolerated.

Whether you side with plaintiffs' lawyers or defendants' lawyers (or are repulsed by the prospect of siding with lawyers at all), this much is clear: The *status* of malpractice litigation is unlikely to remain *quo* for much longer. Politicians are feeling too much pressure to make at least a show of providing constituents with some relief from skyrocketing health care costs. With the recent failure of full-blown health care reform, the courtroom has become the primary target of a scaled-back vision of reform.

TORT REFORM AND
ALTERNATIVE DISPUTE RESOLUTION

Several states have caught tort reform fever. They have taken a variety of measures to bring down the perceived costs, both monetary and non-monetary, of redressing medical negligence. These reforms are the subject of this section of the chapter.

One of the most popular proposals for reforming the malpractice system entails the use of so-called damage caps or liability caps. Caps, where they have been implemented, limit the amount of damages an injured patient can collect in a malpractice suit. With a cap the damages cannot exceed a predetermined limit, regardless of the extent of the patient's injuries.

A fifty-year-old plumber loses his leg as a result of his physician's negligence. The jury awards $1 million. If the liability cap is $500,000, the court will cut the award in half.

Liability caps were included in a package of federal legislation that made some congressional headway in 1995. The measure would have limited punitive damages to $250,000 or three times the amount of actual damages, like lost wages and medical expenses, awarded—whichever was greater. The legislation did not cap actual damages, like lost wages and medical expenses; only punitive damages. The proposal was never enacted into law.

The plaintiffs' bar finds liability caps to be an abomination and a perversion of the judicial system. A fundamental goal of our system of justice is to compensate plaintiffs for the wrong that has been done to them at the hands of the defendant. A jury of the plaintiff's peers is supposed to evaluate the defendant's responsibility, assess the plaintiff's injuries, and award a commensurate sum of damages. Liability caps interrupt this process.

With caps, the amount of damages available to a malpractice plaintiff is preordained by the legislature. Damages are no longer a function of the nature and severity of the plaintiff's injuries and the egregiousness of the defendant's wrongdoing. Instead, damages reflect an arbitrary determination made by lawmakers who are ignorant of the facts and circumstances specific to individual cases.

Advocates of liability caps respond that jury-awarded damages are equally arbitrary. Juries play fast and loose with the insurance companies' money. The typical juror resents wealthy doctors and identifies with injured plaintiffs. He or she becomes overwhelmed with sympathy and generosity, and awards damages that go far beyond what is reasonable.

The idea behind liability caps is to bring down the costs of malpractice litigation by reducing the potential exposure of medical providers. The logic is appealing: Lower damage awards mean malpractice insurers will pay out smaller claims and ultimately save money. Malpractice insurers who save money will reduce their insurance premiums. Doctors who pay reduced insurance premiums will pass the savings on to their patients. Simple as pie.

Or is it? How successful are liability caps at reducing health care costs?

Indiana enacted a total cap on damages in malpractice cases in 1975 (perhaps, not coincidentally, the year Otis Bowen, a physician, served as governor). Despite the caps, health care spending in Indiana increased almost 140 percent between 1980 and 1990, a slightly higher percentage than the national average.

California enacted its Medical Injury Compensation Reform Act (MICRA) in the same year. The act capped non-economic damages at $250,000. Between 1980 and 1989, health care costs in California rose almost 144 percent. Between 1980 and 1986, malpractice premiums for doctors practicing in southern California increased 16 percent for general practitioners and 337 percent for radiologists.[28]

The evidence seems to indicate that liability caps do not reduce health care spending. Why don't they?

First, contrary to popular belief, costs associated with malpractice litigation do not comprise a significant portion of this country's health care expenditures. Malpractice insurance premiums account for less than one percent of the hundreds of billions of dollars the country spends on health care each year.[29] Even if smaller malpractice judgments translated into smaller malpractice insurance premiums, the total impact on health care spending would be minimal.

A second explanation for the apparent failure of caps in controlling health care costs is that insurance companies deny recognizing any cost savings that can be passed along to health care consumers. The caps, if the insurance industry is to be believed, do not limit the insurers' financial outlays. There is reason to view the insurance industry's defense with skepticism. Malpractice insurance carriers enjoy millions of dollars of profits each year.[30]

Third, liability caps do not curtail the costly practice of defensive medicine. Defensive medicine is practiced by doctors who perform unnecessary medical tests and procedures to guard against a charge of negligence. Defensive medicine costs consumers billions of dollars a year—between $15 billion and $40 billion, according to the American Medical Association.[31] It had long been assumed that doctors practice defensive medicine out of fear of a possible claim of malpractice. Now it appears that much of the practice of defensive medicine has nothing to do with malpractice litigation.

Most physicians who order superfluous tests and procedures do so out of ignorance or greed, not fear of legal liability. Some doctors order unnecessary procedures under the mistaken belief that the procedures are medically necessary. Others prescribe superfluous tests to financially enrich themselves because they have a monetary interest in the testing facility. Doctors who partly own testing laboratories have been found to order 34 to 96 percent more tests than doctors without such an investment.[32] Less than 8 percent of unnecessary diagnostic procedures appear to be the result of fear of malpractice.[33]

Liability caps are not the only proposed solution to the alleged malpractice crisis. An alternative reform proposal recommends the domestic adoption of the so-called English Rule. Under the English Rule, whoever loses the lawsuit must pay the winner's attorney fees. In this country, with limited exceptions, both sides pay their own legal fees.

Critics of this proposal, many of whom happen to be lawyers, argue that the English Rule would adversely impact low-income plaintiffs. Poor plaintiffs might be pressured into accepting unreasonably low offers of settlement out of fear of being hit with the other side's legal bill. The existing contingency fee system gives plaintiffs who could not otherwise afford a lawyer access to legal representation.

The English Rule is also arguably superfluous. Losing parties in frivolous U.S. lawsuits can be ordered to pay for the defendant's reasonable attorney fees under existing law. Where a plaintiff brings a case that lacks a minimum degree of merit, the court can direct the plaintiff to compensate the defendant for legal expenses.

Other proposals for reforming the malpractice system do not affect the litigation process itself. Instead, they propose making available alternative methods of resolving malpractice disputes. These alternative methods of resolving malpractice disputes fall under the aptly named rubric *alternative dispute resolution* (ADR). The goal of ADR is to settle claims of malpractice in less time and for less money.

ADR, like ice cream, comes in many flavors. The more popular methods of ADR include the summary jury trial, neutral evaluation, pretrial screening panels, mediation, and arbitration. Each method of ADR, and its proponents and opponents, is considered below.

A summary jury trial is a mini-trial. It has all the trappings of a full-blown trial, including lawyers for both sides, a judge, witnesses, and a jury, but it is missing a key characteristic of the typical jury trial: gross inefficiency. Lawyers are not permitted to argue and argue and argue . . . and then argue some more. They must present their case in four or five hours, and then sit down. Cases that would ordinarily take many weeks to present are concluded within a matter of days. Before the jury comes back with a verdict, counsel for both sides must agree on the maximum amount of damages that can be awarded.

State governments, defense attorneys, and defendants themselves generally like summary jury trials. Public officials are impressed with the way these abbreviated proceedings can clear a crowded court docket. Defense attorneys appreciate the cap on potential damages. Defendants are relieved by the brevity of the proceeding.

Another type of ADR is called neutral evaluation. Neutral evaluation resembles marriage counseling more than it resembles a trial. With neutral evaluation, a disinterested third party hears both sides' stories. The evaluator then decides the relative merit of each side of the case. If the plaintiff's case is weak, the evaluator will try to convince the plaintiff to drop the case. If the plaintiff's case is strong, the evaluator will try to convince the defendant to offer an appropriate settlement. The goal of neutral evaluation is to weed out frivolous cases and resolve meritorious cases as quickly and inexpensively as possible.

Then there is pretrial screening. Pretrial screening works in much the same way as neutral evaluation. The goal of both neutral evaluation and pretrial screening is to cull the strong cases from the weak. However, instead of using a single disinterested party, pretrial screening employs a panel of doctors, lawyers, and laypeople. This panel reviews every malpractice case that is headed for trial. The panel pressures the party with the weaker case to concede defeat or accept a settlement before trial.

About sixteen states mandate pretrial screening. In these states, no malpractice case is heard by a courtroom judge before it is first reviewed by a pretrial screening panel. After review, the screening panel recommends a resolution. The recommendation is just a recommendation; it is not binding on the parties to the dispute. The parties can accept the recommendation and withdraw the legal action, or proceed with the lawsuit. In some state courts, the decisions of screening panels are admissible evidence at the malpractice trial.

Pretrial screening has not enjoyed a problem-free history. Legislators and judges in several states have considered the use of pretrial screening panels, and they have rejected this method of ADR as inefficient or a violation of litigants' right to a speedy trial.

Pretrial screening has been found to be most successful when state law allows the panel's findings to be admitted in a court of law. This rule of evidence discourages parties from trying to take "two bites of the apple" by first going through pretrial screening and then hoping for a better outcome from a trial.

Mediation is not all that different from neutral evaluation. Both types of ADR use a neutral party to help bring the dispute between doctor and patient to an end. The difference is that evaluators try to get rid of bad cases, while mediators try to get defendants to offer settlements that will satisfy even those plaintiffs who have weak cases. Mediators work simultaneously to encourage defendants to propose more generous offers of settlement and to encourage plaintiffs to accept smaller offers of settlement.

Mediation, unlike litigation, is not adversarial. Both sides, with the help of the impartial mediator, are supposed to work together to resolve their disputes. The hope is that by informally searching for a common solution, neither side will suffer the financial and emotional turmoil of a prolonged legal battle. The goal is to keep the anger and rhetoric to a minimum.

Wisconsin is the only state to require mediation before a malpractice case goes to trial. Since 1986, plaintiffs filing a malpractice suit in Wisconsin must submit to mandatory, nonbinding mediation before they file suit or within fifteen days after filing suit. The results have been less than impressive. In 1993, of the 55 percent of plaintiffs who sought mediation before trial, 52 percent proceeded with the lawsuit. Over 55 percent of the plaintiffs who filed for mediation after suing reported that "mediation served no constructive purpose," when polled by the administrator of Wisconsin's Medical Mediation Panels.

Arbitration is the most popular type of ADR. Arbitration is a general term that describes any system whereby one or two neutral outsiders decide the relative guilt and innocence of the parties to the dispute.

Arbitration has both benefits and limitations. Perhaps the primary benefit is a reduction of the time lag between the filing of a complaint and the award of damages. Whereas a malpractice suit typically takes several years to resolve, an arbitration case can be resolved in a matter of months.

A related benefit is the financial savings that are associated with arbitration. Arbitration costs a fraction of the expense of a malpractice trial. Plaintiffs and defendants alike pay dearly to bring and defend malpractice cases.

Arbitrators are also less likely to be swayed by emotion than juries are. Arbitrators are used to hearing tales of woe. They rarely award the types of runaway jury verdicts for pain and suffering that raise the ire of critics of the existing malpractice system. The awards tend to be more compensatory and less punitive.

There is some evidence that the savings that have traditionally been associated with arbitration are disappearing. The arbitration process of today is more complex than that of yesterday. Increasing numbers of plaintiffs come to the arbitration table with legal representation. The attorneys, fearful of sitting like the legendary "potted plant," object to the admission of evidence and often make long-winded arguments in their client's behalf. The longer the proceedings take, the more costly they become.

Arbitration can be voluntary or involuntary, and the verdicts can be binding or nonbinding. In every state, after medical treatment (inside or outside a hospital) has begun, patients and doctors can voluntarily agree to submit to arbitration in the event of a dispute. About fifteen states authorize doctors and patients to agree to voluntary, binding arbitration *before* treatment has begun. A couple of states have made pre-treatment arbitration agreements illegal. (A sample of a voluntary arbitration agreement is reprinted in appendix 5.)

The Clinton administration has thrown its support behind involuntary ("mandatory"), nonbinding arbitration, despite evidence of the inefficacy of this method of ADR. The problem has been that after doctors and patients go through the nonbinding arbitration process, patients who lose the arbitration sue their doctors anyway. The availability of the arbitration only drags out the entire process. Doctors must defend themselves twice, and plaintiffs must wait longer to collect damages.

The Clintons have responded to criticism of their support of nonbinding arbitration by referring to their larger vision of health care reform. If and when universal health care coverage becomes a reality, and every American is guaranteed a basic package of benefits, patients will have less of an incentive to sue for malpractice after the completion of nonbinding arbitration. Their future medical expenses will be covered, so they will not need to chase after larger awards of damages from sympathetic juries.

The Clintons' defense of their position is not universally accepted. They have been accused of supporting nonbinding arbitration because they are lawyers who want other lawyers to like them. Lawyers, as a breed, favor nonbinding arbitration. Nonbinding arbitration protects the legal profession's interest in continuing to bring malpractice lawsuits. The politically influential plaintiffs' bar has been lobbying for nonbinding arbitration for years.

Mandatory binding arbitration has a slightly better reputation, but it is not without its critics. This method of ADR is thought to hamper the informal resolution of doctor-patient disputes. Parties are forced to come together soon after a complaint is filed to attempt to reach an amicable resolution of their differences. Sometimes the parties are not yet ready to deal civilly with each other, and the result is an escalation in antagonism and resistance to settlement.

Michigan is one of the fifteen states that have enacted a voluntary, binding pre-treatment arbitration law. Since the law was passed in 1975, hospitals insured by state-licensed malpractice carriers must offer patients the opportunity to sign agreements consenting to submit any future disputes to arbitration.

Cases that go to arbitration are heard by a three-member panel. The panel is comprised of a medical provider, a lawyer, and a layperson. The arbitration services are purchased from private groups under contract with the state.

A 1990 study conducted by the U.S. General Accounting Office looked at Michigan's experience with voluntary, binding arbitration between 1976 and 1989. The results of the study repudiated some of the perceived benefits of arbitration.

The costs of defending arbitration and litigation malpractice actions were almost the same. While the typical arbitration case cost $17,500 to defend, litigation cost $17,798. There was also not much difference in outcomes from the plaintiffs' perspective. Although the median awards made after arbitration were about $26,000 less than with litigation, plaintiffs prevailed in 3.5 percent more of the arbitration cases. As far as reducing overall malpractice-related costs in the state, arbitration did not have the desired effect. Insurance premiums continued to rise.

There is some evidence that Michigan did not benefit fully from its 1975 enactment because many hospitals avoided the law's reach by self-insuring. There were also legal problems. Lawyers challenged the constitutionality of the statute, and for ten years the issue was debated. Finally, the Michigan Supreme Court upheld the statute, and the lawyers began finding reasons to challenge individual arbitration agreements. Doctors resented having to defend their arbitration agreements from legal attack.

Michigan doctors also disliked asking their patients to sign arbitration agreements before treatment even began. A doctor asking a new patient to sign an arbitration agreement in anticipation of malpractice is like a suitor asking a fiancé to sign a prenuptial agreement in anticipation of a breakup. Neither request fosters feelings of trust or confidence.

Whatever the reasons for its downfall, Michigan lawmakers rescinded the arbitration statute in 1993. The Michigan State Medical Society has recommended a modified version of voluntary, binding arbitration. The society proposes including arbitration provisions in the agreements signed by patients and insurers or managed care programs (such as HMOs). By raising the subject contractually, doctors will not have to discuss the possibility of a malpractice suit directly with their patients, and patients will be more likely to consent to the binding arbitration.

Kaiser Permanente, a huge HMO, already requires most enrollees to take their disputes to binding arbitration. Seventy-eight percent of Kaiser's total membership of almost 7 million enrollees agree to submit their complaints against network providers to binding arbitration. The HMO reports substantial savings on defense costs, and the network providers report a preference for arbitration over litigation.

Unlike the state of Michigan, Kaiser has experienced the promised benefits of arbitration. Kaiser has reported saving $1 million in defense costs alone. In addition, Kaiser has saved money by losing fewer doctor hours to litigation-related business. The HMO found that the arbitration awards compensated injured plaintiffs for their tangible damages but were less likely to include exorbitant damages for pain and suffering.

Plaintiffs' attorneys had concerns about the Kaiser program. They feared that Kaiser was not doing enough to advise enrollees of the full legal implications of the decision to submit to binding arbitration. Enrollees might not understand, for example, that by choosing arbitration they lost the right to call witnesses, present their case to a jury of their peers, and file an appeal.

Kaiser enrollees were also troubled by their HMO's system of arbitration. Although they did win *more* awards with arbitration than with litigation, the size of the arbitration-awarded damages were generally smaller than jury-awarded damages. The enrollees had some concerns that the process was biased against them. The same supposedly neutral arbitrators were repeatedly serving as arbitrators, giving rise to fears of bias. In some states Kaiser was able to mollify enrollees by expanding the pool of neutral arbitrators, but in other states pressure from consumers forced Kaiser to terminate its binding arbitration program.

Kaiser doctors reported a mixed reaction to the use of arbitration. They liked the fact that the average arbitration award was smaller than the average litigation award, but they disliked the fact that they stood a greater chance of losing with arbitration than with litigation. Between 1985 and 1989, the Kaiser enrollees won 52 percent of their arbitration cases and only 25 to 33 percent of their lawsuits.[34]

There are several theories to explain why injured patients win more easily at arbitration than at litigation. Juries might be biased in favor of doctors. They may be more reluctant than arbitrators to find that a doctor has erred (but a jury that finds negligence is quicker than an arbitrator to hit the doctor with hefty damages).

Another theory holds that arbitrators are more Solomonic than judges and juries are. They are more likely to split the proverbial baby in half by awarding *some amount of damages* to the plaintiff, even without proof of medical negligence. They may not grant awards as sizable as a jury would, but they do not like to see plaintiffs walk away from the arbitration table with nothing.

This eagerness to settle cases, with or without proof of the defendant's liability, makes many doctors leery of arbitration. Organized medical professional organizations have not officially supported arbitration. The Health Care Liability Alliance, a tort reform organization that includes the AMA, malpractice insurers, and other health care groups among its members, has not come out in support of arbitration.

ADR has made strange bedfellows of the medical and legal professions. Doctors and lawyers on both sides of malpractice disputes are uniformly skeptical of ADR. Doctors fear that more patients with weaker cases will be making accusations of malpractice and that they will be winning damages. Doctors take small comfort in the fact that the damages awarded with ADR may not be as substantial as those that come with litigation. They still see a threat to their reputation, and a disruption to their professional and personal lives. Lawyers have fears of their own. They worry that the advent of ADR will culminate in the development of a system of dispute resolution that will eventually obliterate the role of lawyers.

RESOURCES

The National Consumers League
815 15th Street, NW
Suite 928-N
Washington, D.C. 20005

Annual membership to The National Consumers League costs $20. The following publications are available for $1.00 each to non-members, and free to members: AIDS: Women at Risk; Guide to Warning Labels on Non-Prescription Medications; Food and Drug Interactions; When Medications Don't Mix: Preventing Drug Interactions; The Pap Test: Assuring Your Good Health; Questions to Ask: Taking Charge of Your Health.

The National Women's Health Network
514 10th Street, N.W., Suite 400
Washington, D.C. 20004
202-347-1140

The National Women's Health Network is a good source of information about abortion and other medical issues of special concern to women. A $25 annual fee entitles members to a subscription to Network News, a bimonthly newsletter, access to the Women's Health Information Service, which is available to answer health care questions, and a discount on network publications.

People's Medical Society
462 Walnut Street
Allentown, PA 18102

The People's Medical Society is a consumer health advocacy organization. The annual membership fee is $20. Members of the society receive a newsletter that suggests ways to get the most out of the health care system, and discounts on numerous publications.

TWO

Your Right of Informed Consent

Does your doctor treat you like you have the mental capacity of a doorknob? Are you reduced to feeling like a schoolchild by the time you leave your doctor's office?

If you answer these questions in the affirmative, you're not alone. Many patients credit their doctors with a superiority complex. They fault their doctors for acting as if patients are incapable of understanding the nature of their medical condition, appreciating their treatment options, and making informed decisions regarding their care.

The result can be a vicious Catch-22.

The process starts with a doctor who doesn't perceive a patient to be capable of participating in treatment decisions. The doctor withholds from the patient the very information the patient needs to make knowledgeable health care decisions. Deprived of this information, the patient cannot ask appropriate and intelligent questions regarding the nature of his or her illness and treatment options. Attempts by the patient to formulate questions come out sounding awkward and confused. Patient fumphering, in turn, affirms the doctor's perception of the patient's ignorance, and justifies the further withholding of information.

Doctors are under a legal obligation to talk to their patients. They must provide their patients with enough information about the patient's medical condition and treatment options to enable the patient to make an informed decision about whether or not to consent to a proposed test or procedure. Doctors who treat patients without first obtaining the patient's informed consent to the intended treatment are breaking the law.

Although some doctors are guilty of sabotaging communications with patients, others take the time to explain, in complete and easy-to-understand language, what the patient needs to know about his or her prognosis and care. These doctors appreciate the patient's capacity to understand medical concepts and participate in the formulation of a treatment plan. Questions from patients are welcomed, not feared as a threat to the doctor's authority.

Some communication gap between doctors and patients may be unavoidable. Doctors speak their own language. The technical terms they use to describe medical conditions, treatments, and outcomes with specificity and exactitude cannot easily be translated into plain English. A degree of precision is inevitably lost when lay language replaces medical terminology. The gap only widens in breadth when the patient speaks a different language or has minimal education.

Some patients resist taking a role in directing the course of their care. They prefer to leave medical decision making to their doctors. For these patients, frank and open discussions about the pros and cons of chemotherapy versus radiation therapy, drugs versus surgery, or in-patient versus out-patient care only serve to increase their anxiety.

Dr. Franz Ingelfinger, a former editor of *The New England Journal of Medicine*, was one such patient. When Dr. Ingelfinger fell ill, his medical colleagues bombarded him with a wealth of information about the relative risks and benefits of alternative treatments. He soon became confused and distraught, and sought the counsel of a trusted physician friend. The friend told him, "You need a doctor." Dr. Ingelfinger took this advice to mean that he should find someone who would tell him what to do and assume total responsibility for his care. He did, and experienced an immediate sense of relief.

Doctors who give their patients too much information are sometimes accused of "truth dumping." Truth dumping leaves patients confused, not informed.

It is not always easy for a doctor to know how much information is too much. Thanks to advances in medical technology, doctors now have access to tremendous amounts of information about almost every ailment. The disclosure of this information forces patients to make difficult, if not impossible, medical choices. A few examples illustrate the problem.

➤ A pregnant woman goes in for a sonogram, which reveals that the baby's urinary system is blocked. The doctors advise the woman that the baby could be born normal, might require dialysis or an organ transplant, or will die shortly after birth. The woman and her husband must decide whether to abort the fetus or proceed with the pregnancy.

➤ When a thirty-six-year-old stockbroker is diagnosed with cancer of the lymph nodes, his doctors give him three options: Open heart surgery, chemotherapy, or a bone marrow transplant. He learns that the cancerous tumor would be more likely to return after surgery or chemotherapy, but the transplant could cause life-threatening bouts of anemia, bleeding, infection, and pain. The ultimate decision about which course to pursue rests solely on his shoulders.

➤ A middle-aged woman experiencing fatigue is diagnosed with a weakening of the heart. She is advised that medication might slow down the deterioration of her heart muscle, but would not cure her. A heart transplant, if successful, could add years to her life, but five percent of all transplant patients die within a month of surgery. She has to grapple with the decision for months.

Even patients who want to know everything about their condition and care may not want to know a doctor's best guess at their life expectancy. Should doctors tell terminally ill patients how long they are likely to live? The question is a difficult one to answer, as the following case demonstrates.

A patient was undergoing kidney surgery when his surgeons discovered and removed a cancerous tumor from his pancreas. The surgeon referred the patient to a specialist, but he did not inform him that pancreatic cancer spreads quickly and only five percent of patients diagnosed with pancreatic cancer survive five years.

At their first meeting, the specialist asked the patient how much the patient wanted to know about his illness. The patient responded that he wanted to know the truth.

The specialist prescribed radiation and chemotherapy treatments, and advised the patient that the treatments might prevent recurrence or might be completely ineffective. When test results showed that the cancer had apparently recurred, the specialist did not tell the patient that his reasonable life expectancy could be measured in months. Two months later, when the patient was hospitalized, the specialist told the patient that he could not be cured but "they could try to make things better so that he might have some good time ahead." The patient died the following month.

The patient's wife and children sued the surgeon and the specialist. They charged the doctors with breaching their duty to disclose material information by failing to tell the patient his life expectancy. They claimed that the patient might have opted against the time-consuming and painful treatments, and might have redone his Last Will and Testament, if he had known he had only a couple of months to live.

Did the doctors provide the patient with enough information to make informed decisions regarding his care? If so, was that enough? Or did the patient have a fundamental right to know how long he had to live? Most judges, when confronted with these difficult questions, come down in favor of requiring disclosure of statistical information about life expectancy. A study conducted at the George

Washington University Medical Center in Washington, D.C., found that most patients want to know when they are going to die.

The question of how much people want to know about their life expectancy is becoming less and less academic. Researchers have now developed a computer program that can predict with 82 percent accuracy whether a patient is going to die within six months. The program can also make a month-to-month prediction of the likelihood of death.[35]

The standard for physician disclosure has not always been the same. The following section explores informed consent, both past and present. The discussion is followed by a look at informed consent in the context of medical research, testing for the AIDS virus, medical malpractice, medical screening, treatment of minors, and abortion. The chapter concludes with a brief consideration of economic informed consent, which limits the physician's duty of disclosure when the patient lacks the financial resources to afford every available treatment.

HISTORICAL OVERVIEW

The right of informed consent as a legal concept derives from the right to be free of unwanted touching. Since the early 1900s, the courts determined that when one individual touches another individual without the second individual's consent, there is a criminal assault and battery, regardless of the toucher's profession. Doctors were given no special touching privileges. To date, a doctor is not permitted to touch a patient, or anyone else for that matter, without that person's consent, for therapeutic purposes or otherwise.

Over time, the assault and battery rationale for requiring doctors to disclose information to their patients so that their patients would consent to be touched was replaced by a more general duty of disclosure. The general duty of disclosure was premised on the inequality of doctors and patients. Doctors are strong; patients are vulnerable. Doctors are informed; patients are ignorant. Courts imposed on doctors a duty to care for their dependent patients.

This duty of care entailed informing patients about the nature and consequences of proposed tests and treatments, and obtaining the patient's consent. Doctors who failed to fulfill this duty were guilty of civil negligence, not criminal assault and battery.

Physicians faced greater legal exposure as the assault and battery theory of liability gave way to the negligence theory. A physician who failed to advise his patient of the risks of forgoing a Pap smear, for example, would not be liable for assault and battery. There is no assault and battery in the absence of physical contact, or the threat of contact, between doctor and patient. Such a physician would, however, face potential liability for negligence. The doctor would have breached his duty by withholding information that his patient needed in order to make a knowledgeable decision about her medical care.

In the late 1950s, the courts expanded the scope of mandatory disclosure. Not only were doctors duty-bound to disclose information about a proposed test or treatment but they also became obligated to provide information about alternative treatments. The idea that patients could give informed consent to a proposed procedure only if they knew the risks and benefits of their treatment options achieved legal recognition.

The standard of what constitutes adequate disclosure has changed over time. In the past, doctors fulfilled their duty of disclosure by telling their patients whatever information a "reasonable physician" would disclose under similar circumstances. A physician who reasonably believed that the patient only needed to know X, Y, and Z, and disclosed only these three facts, met his duty of disclosure.

Over time, however, the courts began requiring doctors to disclose the information a "reasonable patient" would want to be told under similar circumstances. Doctors could no longer base their disclosures on what the doctor believed the patient needed to know. The courts wanted the doctors to stand in their patients' shoes, and consider what their patients would want to know given the prevailing conditions.

The changing standard of disclosure made physicians edgy. They were unsure of what was required of them, and they asked state legislatures to clarify the rules governing informed consent.

Before long, state informed consent statutes started appearing on law books across the country. Today the statutory standard of disclosure varies from state to state.

Some states have adopted the professional standard, which requires disclosure of the information a reasonable doctor believes necessary. Other jurisdictions have incorporated the patient-based standard. A minority of specific informed consent statutes spell out precisely what information must be provided to patients considering specific medical procedures, such as electroconvulsive therapy, sterilization, breast cancer therapies, and abortion.

On the federal level, the National Childhood Vaccination Compensation Injury Act requires physicians who administer certain immunizations to provide their patients with informational booklets. The booklets, which were developed by the national Centers for Disease Control, explain possible reactions to the vaccine, contraindications, and recommended schedules for administration. Patients must be provided with these booklets as part of the informed consent process.

To say that a doctor must disclose what a reasonable physician or reasonable patient would disclose or want to be disclosed under similar circumstances is reasonably confusing to any reasonable person. Use the criteria listed below to determine whether you are in a position to give informed consent to a proposed medical procedure. A sample consent form is reprinted in appendix 6.

➤ *Are you informed?* To be informed, you must have had an opportunity to discuss with your doctor, or any knowledgeable health care provider, the history of your medical condition, the nature and purpose of the proposed procedure, attendant risks of the proposed procedure, the possibility of success, your prognosis if the procedure is not performed, and the benefits and limitations of available treatment alternatives. Anticipated costs of treatment and possible effects on your lifestyle, such as mobility limitations, dietary restrictions, and ongoing monitoring requirements, should also be discussed. If your doctor proposes a new medication regimen, you should be told why the medication is needed, why the prescription is being changed, possible side effects, and the availability and advantages of surgical and nonsurgical alternatives.

➤ *Do you understand the information that has been provided to you?* Your consent will not be valid, regardless of what your doctor tells you, if you did not comprehend the information provided to you. Doctors who routinely use five-syllable words to explain medical concepts to patients who did not graduate sixth grade, or who speak English to their Spanish-speaking patients, do not meet their duty of disclosure.

➤ *Is your consent voluntary?* Consent that is obtained through the use of coercion or undue influence is invalid. For example, a doctor who leads a patient to believe that she must consent to a medical procedure or risk an immediate hospital discharge taints the legality of the patient's consent. Similarly, a surgeon who intimidates a patient into consenting to a treatment by questioning her sanity if she refuses the recommended course of care may not obtain valid consent.

➤ *Are you competent to give consent?* A patient who is so mentally or physically incapacitated that he or she has lost the ability to make decisions about care cannot give informed consent. Decision-making capability, at a minimum, entails an ability to understand and appreciate what the proposed treatment involves and its possible consequences. Any reasoned decision you make must be consistent with your own values and beliefs. Your reasoned decisions must be respected, even if others consider your decision to be off-the-wall. A fully competent patient can rationally decide not to undergo a treatment that everyone else, including her doctor, spouse, and children, thinks she should undergo. (The rules that govern medical decision making by patients who lack the capacity to make decisions for themselves are covered in depth in chapter 6.)

When a patient refuses to consent to a recommended medical treatment, questions about the patient's competence usually follow in short stead. Doctors are concerned about their legal exposure. There have been cases in which physicians who comply with an incompetent patient's refusal to consent to a recommended treatment are found guilty of negligence.

Doctors who are called upon to make a determination of competency must do a careful balancing of the patient's right to self-determination and the physician's own professional responsibility to provide appropriate medical care. The courts have instructed doctors to find competent those patients who are capable of appreciating their medical condition and the risks of forgoing treatment.

The difficulty of applying this nebulous standard in practice is well illustrated by two cases. In one case, a delusional patient with schizophrenia was found competent to withhold consent to breast cancer surgery because she could express a desire to have her body remain intact.[36] In the second case, a delusional schizophrenic man was found incompetent to withhold consent to life-saving surgery when he could not communicate an understanding of the risk of death.[37] The fact that the determination of competency must often be made under conditions of urgency and anxiety leaves the process even more vulnerable to error.

If a determination is being made that you or someone you love is not competent to withhold consent to treatment, here are some questions to ask. The more questions that are answered in the affirmative, the stronger is the case for proving competency.

➤ Can the patient label her illness?

➤ Does the patient connect her illness to her presence in the medical facility?

➤ Can the patient describe the nature of the recommended procedure?

➤ Can the patient explain the purpose of the recommended procedure?

➤ Can the patient state risks associated with the recommended procedure?

➤ Can the patient give reasons for her decision to withhold consent?

➤ Can the patient name alternative treatments?

➤ Does the patient express an understanding of the consequences of receiving no treatment?

➤ Has the patient consistently withheld consent, rather than waffle back and forth between withholding and granting consent?

The rule of informed consent, like every rule, has exceptions. One exception applies to emergency treatment. In an emergency, doctors may do that which is necessary to preserve life and limb without the patient's consent. This exception is premised on the theory of implied consent. Incapacitated patients in emergency situations who are facing imminent harm are presumed to consent to emergency care, in the absence of an advance directive providing otherwise. (See chapter 6 for discussion of advance directives.)

A second exception to the informed consent requirement applies where the interests of society are involved. A mass inoculation program to protect the public's health, for example, will be carried out without obtaining each individual's consent.

The third and final exception permits doctors to withhold information from their patients if disclosure would harm the patient. This exception is often referred to as the "therapeutic privilege." The scope of this exception varies somewhat from state to state. In some jurisdictions, doctors are permitted to withhold information if disclosure would cause any deterioration in the patient's physical or mental condition. Other jurisdictions allow nondisclosure only in those situations where disclosure would jeopardize treatment. Doctors are never permitted to rely on the therapeutic privilege to overcome a patient's reluctance to undergo a recommended treatment.

Informed consent is an ongoing process of communication between doctors and patients. It is not a one-shot deal where the doctor gives the patient some information and the patient gives the doctor a thumbs-up or thumbs-down. The health care provider must be available to the patient to answer questions, review or supplement previously discussed information, and negotiate and amend treatment plans. The patient's signature on a consent form is supposed to indicate that the entire informed consent process has taken place.

Some doctors delegate their duty of disclosure. They send an attending nurse to the patient's room with instructions to get the patient's signature on a general consent form. If anything goes wrong, a doctor who obtained the patient's consent in this manner may well be liable for breaching the doctor's non-delegable legal duty to educate the patient. Primary responsibility for informing patients about the nature and purpose of proposed medical procedures, and the risks and benefits of alternative treatments, rests with the physician who ordered or performed the procedure.

In certain limited cases, nurses are charged with the primary duty of disclosure. As health care professionals, nurses have assumed greater autonomy over time. When a nurse acts independently in evaluating the risks and benefits of a certain medical procedure, the nurse may be legally charged with primary responsibility for obtaining the patient's informed consent. Especially in the home care setting, where nurses exercise a high degree of autonomy, the duty of disclosure may rest with a nurse.

RIGHTS OF MEDICAL RESEARCH SUBJECTS

Medical research has a gruesome past, but a glorious present and future. Decades ago, participants in medical research were often ignorant of the dangers they faced. Their suffering led to the development of strict guidelines of research ethics. These guidelines protect research subjects of today.

Participants in medical research must now be adequately informed of the aims, methods, anticipated benefits, and potential hazards of the study and the discomforts it may entail. They must have sufficient knowledge and comprehension of the nature, purpose, possible effects, and methods of the study to make an enlightened decision about participation.

Researchers must tell prospective subjects the purpose of the study, the anticipated duration, the risks, benefits, and potential costs of participation, and the availability of compensation in the event of a mishap. Participants must sign a form indicating that they have received the required information, understand the risks and benefits of participation, and have consented to participate freely, without the intervention of any element of force or fraud.

These requirements, and more, are set forth in the Nuremberg Code, Declaration of Helsinki, federal regulations, and in state statutes.

Now, thanks in large part to discoveries made during clinical trials, about 90 percent of children with leukemia, Hodgkin's disease, and Wilms' tumor can be cured. Women with breast cancer who once faced disfiguring surgery or death are now successfully treated with less invasive surgery, chemotherapy, and radiation therapy. The discovery of the effectiveness of aspirin against strokes, AZT against AIDS, cholesterol-reducing clofibrate against heart attacks, and vaccines against polio, measles, and rubella are all the fruit of past medical research.

Clinical trials test the safety and effectiveness of new therapies and treatments. Clinicians systematically study patients to compare the relative costs and benefits of new and standard approaches to particular medical conditions.

Just about every clinical trial is designed to answer the same question: Which treatment is better—the new or the old? A look at the research that is currently being conducted to find a pharmaceutical treatment for Alzheimer's disease shows how a typical clinical trial works.

The first step in any clinical trial is for researchers to determine that the drug that is the subject of the study is safe for testing on humans. After this initial determination of safety is made, a preliminary trial is commenced. This trial involves only a small number of patients and healthy volunteers. The purpose of the preliminary trial is to learn about dosage levels, side effects, and the general safety of the drug.

If everything looks good after the preliminary trial, the researchers can begin the clinical trial itself. The purpose of the clinical trial is to determine the drug's treatment potential, and to learn more about the effect of the drug on the human body.

The clinical trial involves the administration of the drug to some patients, and administration of a placebo to others. The placebo looks just like the real drug but has absolutely no effect on the body. The pills are coded. Even the doctors conducting the study do not know which pills are the real McCoy and which are dummies.

When the study is concluded, the results are analyzed. If the drug is found to have a positive effect in controlling the symptoms of Alzheimer's, patients in the trial may be allowed to use the drug.

Patients who join a clinical trial stand to benefit from a promising new treatment. That's an inducement to participate. There are, however, deterrents to participation. The patient may be unwilling to play the role of human guinea pig. Or perhaps the patient's doctor is pressuring the patient not to participate so that the doctor can retain primary control over the patient.

Patients are not allowed to participate in clinical studies without first giving their voluntary informed consent. If the patient lacks the mental capacity to consent, a family member with legal authority to act on the patient's behalf will be able to give consent on the patient's behalf.

If you or someone you represent is considering participation in a clinical trial, be sure to:

➤ Find out all you can about the nature and purpose of the study. The researchers should be willing to provide you with complete answers to the following questions: What are the potential risks and benefits of the alternative treatments? What information exists regarding the efficacy of the procedures or drugs being studied? How can you gain access to that information, and who will help you understand the information? What other similar studies have been performed?

➤ Ask questions about the design of the study. Are different treatments assigned to participants at random? Will your request for a particular treatment be accommodated? If the different treatments are randomly assigned to participants, you should withhold consent unless and until you are convinced that each treatment under study offers comparable risks and benefits.

➤ Carefully review the informed consent form. The researchers should be willing to go over every word on the form. The form should explain that the treatment under study is experimental, and it should list any known possible side effects. The purpose of the study should also be explained in plain English. Make sure that you will have opportunities for further discussions with knowledgeable health care professionals if questions arise. Inquire about the procedures for withdrawing consent.

➤ Refuse to sign anything that waives your rights in the event the patient is harmed during the study.

➤ Be suspicious about any fees associated with the study. Participants in medical research are not usually asked to pay for the experimental drug.

➤ Verify that the Food and Drug Administration (FDA) has approved the study.

➤ Ask if an open label extension is part of the study. After the completion of an open label study, the patient can opt to continue receiving the drug for a specified period of time.

Some medical ethicists believe that obtaining voluntary informed consent to some types of medical research is an impossibility. Seriously ill patients, these ethicists argue, are under such intense pressures that they are not in any position to rationally balance the risks and benefits of participating in a clinical trial. They agree to participate in the research for reasons that have nothing to do with a well-reasoned analysis of the medical risks and benefits of participation. Fear, economic concerns, and family pressures leave many patients incapable of making a rational decision about participation.

Many patients enroll in medical studies just to accommodate their doctors. Their consent reflects their eagerness to please their doctor, to whom they often feel a debt of gratitude. They feel compelled to accede to their physician's urgings to join the study and are unwilling to risk antagonizing their doctor by challenging the contents of the consent form.

Rigorous informed consent requirements raise some practical difficulties for doctors and researchers. Take, for example, the study of alternative cancer treatments. In a nationwide clinical trial that compared breast cancer treatments, few women were willing to undergo a mutilating radical mastectomy once they learned that less invasive alternative treatments were available.

Some medical researchers theorize that the slow progress that has been made over the past twenty years in treating cancers of the lung, breast, colon, and prostate is attributable to the reluctance of potential research subjects to participate in clinical trials. Less than 2 percent of all adults with common forms of cancer participate in clinical trials. Interestingly, about 70 percent of all children with cancer participate in clinical trials, and relatively more treatment methods have been developed for childhood cancers.[38]

In addition to the practical difficulties associated with informed consent and medical research, the process has the potential to destroy a doctor-patient relationship. Take, for example, a study of alternative cervical cancer treatments.

The conventional treatment for cancer of the cervix over the past fifty years has been radiotherapy; medical researchers then discover a chemical agent that shows potential for increasing cure rates when used with radiotherapy. They commence a clinical trial. The researchers recruit a doctor to find qualified research subjects. He identifies a patient as a potential participant. He calls the patient into his office to explain the purpose of the study. The patient, impressed with the potential benefit of the newly discovered chemotherapy treatment, agrees to participate in the study.

The researchers conducting the study randomly select the patient to receive radiotherapy alone. The patient, distressed by the prospect of losing out on the promising experimental treatment, confronts her doctor. The doctor, in a well-meaning effort to comfort his patient, minimizes the promise of the chemotherapy.

The result is bad all around. The patient is left feeling deceived and cheated of the best possible care. The physician comes off looking like a charlatan who had either hyped the experimental treatment to gain the patient's consent, or lied about the comparable efficacy of the two treatments. The doctor is left in a lose-lose situation.

The problems that attend the informed consent process are heightened when the subject of the research is alcohol, drug abuse, incest, family violence, or some other socially unacceptable or illegal practice. Once the subject matter of the study is disclosed to potential participants, the likelihood of voluntary participation drops dramatically. Promises of confidentiality and anonymity fall silently on ears deafened by fears of public embarrassment and legal recriminations. From the researcher's perspective, the result is a study threatened with bias from the get-go.

Studies of stigmatizing behavior are tainted even further because test subjects are inclined to lie. Researchers studying substance abuse, for example, expect a certain percentage of subjects to minimize the extent of their drug use to protect themselves. Understandably, researchers conducting such studies like to independently verify the information being provided to them. In a study of drug use, for example, the researchers may want to test body fluids to verify information provided by the patient.

But there's a hitch. Investigators cannot collect blood or urine samples from study participants without first disclosing the uses to which the samples will be put. The subjects must be told that the samples will be tested to identify those who lie to the researchers. Since no one will want to be caught in a lie, the subjects will alter their behavior in anticipation of the testing program, or they will withhold their consent to the tests. The value of the independent testing will plummet.

What should a researcher do when presented with such a quandary: Accept the skewed test results or proceed without obtaining the subjects' informed consent?

Investigators who have resolved this dilemma by conducting their studies without getting their subjects' informed consent justify their violation of the canons of research ethics. They argue that research into deviant behavior is essential to the development of sound social policy and cannot be abandoned. They further argue that the interests of the test subjects are adequately protected as long as any possible link between an individual subject and the data collected is destroyed.

This balancing of the benefit of research with the cost to the subject is not enough to justify conducting a study without informed consent, according to many medical ethicists. Potential test subjects must be given the opportunity to refuse to participate in the study, even if their refusal is unreasonable or thwarts the development of social policy. Strict adherence to the requirements of informed consent is necessary to protect the personal autonomy of test subjects. The danger of abuse is too substantial to allow exceptions.

At least to some extent, this issue may soon be addressed by federal legislation. In 1995 a U.S. congressman proposed legislation that included a mandatory parental consent requirement for social research into the behaviors of American teens. The bill required parents to give written consent before their children could be questioned in a federally funded study about sexual behavior or "illegal, antisocial or self-incriminating behavior."

In introducing the legislation, the congressman expressed his dismay at learning that his two high school–age children had been questioned about their virginity and use of contraceptives as part of a federally funded study. Traditionally, researchers studying drinking, drugs, smoking, and sex among teens usually gave parents the opportunity to object to their children's participation, either over the telephone or in a letter. The new legislation explicitly required the parents' written consent. To date, the bill has not yet been signed into law.

Social researchers oppose mandatory parental consent. They say the new consent process will be costly, adding about 50 percent to the cost of the research, and will skew the test results. Low-income and minority parents statistically have a lower response rate. In one inner-city Michigan school, only 17 out of 100 parents returned the consent form. As a result, poor and minority children will be underrepresented in the studies.[39]

When investigators do not meet the letter and spirit of their informed consent obligations, whether out of a selfish eagerness to advance their research goals, or zeal to make a discovery to benefit society, or honest ignorance, the results can be devastating. The National Institutes of Health (NIH) issued a report in March 1994 that described how researchers at the University of California, Los Angeles, had failed to obtain proper consent from people who participated in a study of how schizophrenics coped with the termination of antipsychotic drugs.

About half of the participants in the schizophrenia study suffered severe relapses after being taken off their medication. One participant committed suicide, another broke his back in a suicide attempt, and three others suffered permanent mental damage from their relapses. The Federal Office of Protection from Research Risks found that the consent forms the patients signed did not adequately describe the potential magnitude of the relapses. The government agency concluded that the study was unethical and violated federal regulations because the subjects had not been adequately informed about the risks of participation.[40]

Existing informed consent guidelines do not offer specific guidance to doctors who stand to benefit financially from their involvement in medical research. This issue is of fairly recent origin. The question that has arisen is whether doctors must disclose their financial interests to their patients.

Imagine, for example, that a surgeon is working with a biotechnology company on a discovery that could make the doctor a millionaire. Sometimes, when the doctor is performing an operation, he removes a small sample of tissue from his patient to advance his biotechnology research. The removal of the tissue sample does not cause the patient any pain, and does not adversely affect the patient's health.

Is the doctor in this example obligated to tell his patients that he intends to use their tissue in connection with a potentially lucrative research project? Or do patients relinquish ownership of their body parts when they consent to the surgery? Since the removal of the tissue sample does not involve any risks or benefits to the patient, why should additional consent be required?

Those who favor disclosure argue that a patient should be able to consent to surgery without losing any fundamental control over his or her body parts. The removal of the tissue samples, the argument goes, is a separate medical procedure that requires independent disclosure and consent. The existence or nonexistence of potential harm to the patient is irrelevant. Furthermore, patients assume their doctors are solely accountable to them. The patient pays the doctor a fee, and the doctor treats the patient. If the doctor also has some other allegiance, say to a research company, the patient has a right to know that the situation is not as he or she assumes it to be.

Financial disclosure to patients is not required by guidelines prepared by the U.S. Department of Health and Human Services, the American Federation of Clinical Research, or the American College of Physicians. The American Medical Association's Council on Ethical and Judicial Affairs has taken the position that conflicts between a physician's financial interests and a patient's benefit should be resolved in favor of the patient, but it has not recommended the disclosure of financial interests by physicians to patients.

Pharmaceutical companies use doctors to research new drugs in ways that raise additional concerns about financial disclosure and informed consent. Some doctors are on the payroll of drug manufacturers. Drug companies pay the doctors to prepare and file reports concerning their patients' response to drugs that have recently been approved for sale by the Food and Drug Administration (FDA). The practice is commonly known by a name worthy of a *Star Trek* episode—Phase IV research. The goal of Phase IV research is to uncover unanticipated side effects and to determine appropriate dosages of new pharmaceuticals.

When patients are asked to consent to participate in Phase IV testing, they are told that the testing is part of a pharmaceutical company's post-marketing research. They may also be given financial inducements, such as free medication, tests, and office visits. They are rarely, however, told that the pharmaceutical company is paying their physician for each patient the doctor enrolls in the study. That information would come as a surprise to many Phase IV participants.

The physician's financial stake in Phase IV research creates a potential conflict of interest. A doctor is supposed to make decisions about prescription medications based solely on the patient's therapeutic needs. When a pharmaceutical company offers the doctor a financial incentive to prescribe a recently approved medication instead of a well-established competitor, there is a clear danger that the doctor's prescribing practices will be unduly influenced.

Research into new resuscitation procedures (restarting the heartbeat or respiration) raises different, but equally troubling, issues. Although prior informed consent of participants is required for resuscitation research, as for any other type of medical research, resuscitation researchers can rarely obtain their subjects' consent. A potential subject who suddenly stops breathing after a trauma to the head or drug overdose cannot be expected to say her name, much less give informed consent to an experimental resuscitation technique.

Most doctors in such a situation have traditionally given randomly selected patients the experimental treatment, or used the experimental procedure to try to save the lives of patients only where no standard treatment is available or no reasonable and competent patient would refuse the experimental treatment, or they have used the experimental treatment without the patient's consent since obtaining truly informed consent under the circumstances is an impossibility and the public has an overriding interest in the development of new resuscitation techniques. Although these theories have influenced decisions about resuscitation research for years, none has been incorporated in the relevant federal regulations.[41]

In September 1995 the Food and Drug Administration proposed rules to make it easier to perform experimental medical treatments on patients who are unable to give their consent, either because they are unconscious or in the midst of a medical emergency. The commissioner, in proposing the rules, conceded that the existing regulations were conflicting and confusing and discouraged experimentation when the patient's informed consent could not be obtained.

Under the new rules, experiments in emergency settings would be allowed if other available treatments are unproved or unsatisfactory, the patient is in a life-threatening situation, researchers cannot obtain the information any other way, and the risks and benefits are in reasonable balance in light of other possible treatments. The proposed rules are expected to take effect after a forty-five-day period of public comment.

In the beginning of 1995, doctors, scientists, and medical ethicists convened in Baltimore to discuss medical research and informed consent. A consensus emerged that the existing system could benefit from reform.[42]

Suggestions for reform included inviting patient and consumer advocates to join the institutional review boards that review experiment proposals at research institutions; having third parties question research subjects to make sure consent is both voluntary and informed; and requiring medical facilities to include monitoring of research projects in their quality control program. Some participants at the meeting also wanted to see the federal government establish a national human experimentation board to oversee the 4,000 independent institutional review boards that exist across the country. Although the meeting was characterized by divergent opinions, everyone agreed that the existing consent forms are technical and of little use to patients.

Most patients learn about opportunities to participate in medical research from their physicians. If you are interested in learning about trials of experimental treatments that may be beneficial to you, the first place to start is with your doctor. It is best if your doctor makes inquiries into pending clinical studies on your behalf.

If your physician is not helpful or informed, you should contact the national organization that is concerned with the disease in question (such as the Alzheimer's Association) or the National Institutes of Health in Bethesda, Maryland, to get the names of doctors and medical centers in your area that are conducting relevant clinical trials. Occasionally you may see an advertisement for research volunteers in a local newspaper. (Advocacy organizations listed by disease or disability appear in appendix 7.)

You can learn about cancer research projects by calling The National Cancer Institute's Cancer Information Service at 1-800-4-CANCER (422-6237). The institute provides information about clinical trials directly to the public. For information specifically about medical research into childhood cancers, contact the Candelighters Childhood Cancer Foundation, 7910 Woodmont Avenue, Bethesda, MD 20814; telephone number 301-657-8401.

LEGAL REQUIREMENTS OF TESTING FOR AIDS

The issue of informed consent and HIV and AIDS testing has been hotly contested in recent years by judges, legislators, and the public. The competing rights and interests are difficult to reconcile. The public's interest in controlling the devastating AIDS epidemic must be carefully balanced with the public's expectation of privacy with respect to personal medical matters.

Perhaps the best place to begin an examination of this multifarious issue is with the American Medical Association (AMA). The AMA's internally inconsistent position on patient consent and testing for the human immunodeficiency virus (HIV)—the virus that causes AIDS—reflects the complexity of the problem.

In December 1991, the AMA's House of Delegates adopted a policy that allowed HIV testing without explicit informed consent from the patient. Simple enough, except the policy conflicted with the AMA's own ethics code. In a 1992 opinion prepared by the Council on Ethical and Judicial Affairs, the AMA stated, "Physicians should ensure that HIV testing is conducted in a way that respects patient autonomy and assures patient confidentiality as much as possible. The physician should secure the patient's informed consent specific for HIV testing before testing is performed." [43]

Eventually the conflict was resolved in favor of the council. The council was found to impose a higher obligation on physicians than the House of Delegates.

AMA members who favor the council's position defend the requirement of informed consent on several grounds. First, patients have a fundamental right to control what is done to their bodies. Testing without explicit and informed consent defiles that right. Furthermore, the process of obtaining informed consent serves an educational function. The patient receives important information about the nature of the HIV virus, and counseling about the consequences of HIV infection. Patients who undergo this process are better prepared for the test results.

Some states have passed laws that apply specifically to HIV testing. At the time of publication, thirty-eight states require informed consent for HIV testing, twenty-two allow testing without consent for emergency care or if the patient is unable to give consent, and thirty states allow testing without consent if health care workers or emergency personnel have been exposed to HIV.

An Alabama law allowed HIV testing without the patient's written informed consent if the patient was at high risk for infection based on a physician's "reasonable medical judgment." A federal judge found that nonconsensual HIV testing based on a physician's perception of the patient's risk of infection violated the equal protection clause of the U.S. Constitution. The law created a distinct class of people—those considered to be at high risk for HIV infection—and then treated them differently by allowing them to be tested without their consent, which is unconstitutional.[44]

Nonconsensual testing of patients suspected of HIV infection was also found by the judge in the Alabama case to risk enhancing the spread of AIDS. The court expressed concern that high-risk individuals might avoid seeking medical attention if they feared being tested for HIV infection against their will. Individuals given the opportunity to voluntarily submit to HIV testing might be more inclined to seek counseling and treatment.

Now HIV testing without the subject's written, informed consent is legal in Alabama under two limited circumstances: when it is necessary to protect the safety and well-being of health care workers, and if knowledge of the patient's HIV status would affect the course of treatment selected.

The judge's decision to allow nonconsensual testing under these two limited exceptions angered advocates on both sides of the dispute. Those opposed to involuntary testing argued that nonconsensual testing is never justified, under any circumstances. Those who favored destigmatizing AIDS by treating it like any other infectious disease for which testing without consent is allowed were also disappointed.

Even where state law does not allow nonconsensual testing based on the physician's perceived risk of infection, there remains a potential for discriminatory testing. Take, for example, state statutes that allow testing without consent based on "medical necessity." Many of these statutes fail to define what constitutes medical necessity. Doctors who favor widespread testing can justify greater instances of medical necessity than do those who oppose the testing.

The recently developed S.U.D.S. (Single Use Diagnostic System) HIV-1 Test poses a new threat to the patient's right of informed consent. On one level, the S.U.D.S. test has everything going for it. It's fast (results within ten minutes), easy (requires only minimal training), inexpensive (under $10 each) and accurate (over 99 percent). The S.U.D.S. test received FDA approval in 1992.

Anxious patients whose fears of HIV infection are unwarranted could not ask for a test better suited to their needs. There is some fear, however, that S.U.D.S. tests will be performed without the patient's consent, even though the same consent requirements apply to S.U.D.S. that apply to traditional HIV diagnostic testing. The S.U.D.S. test can be performed in a doctor's office or clinic, unlike other tests, which must be performed at laboratory testing centers. The S.U.D.S. test also yields results within minutes, unlike other tests, which can take days or even weeks.

Testing for HIV infection without the patient's consent raises a number of concerns. First and foremost, nonconsensual testing violates the patient's autonomy. Second, doctors may use the test results to deny treatment to patients who test positive, even though refusing to treat someone because of HIV infection is legally and ethically wrong under most circumstances. Finally, patients who are tested without their consent are less likely to receive the appropriate pre- and post-test counseling.

MEDICAL MALPRACTICE AND NONDISCLOSURE

Most state laws on medical malpractice incorporate some type of informed consent provisions. Typically these provisions require physicians licensed in the state to disclose to their patients the information necessary to enable a reasonable person under similar circumstances to intelligently consent to, or refuse, a proposed treatment. In some jurisdictions, doctors have been excused from discussing detailed technical medical concepts that the patient is unlikely to understand. In other jurisdictions, doctors are not required to advise their patients of remote risks and side effects. Sometimes doctors are given discretion to withhold potentially frightening information that would undermine a patient's rationality and decision-making ability.

Judges hearing these types of cases do not have an easy job. They must distinguish cases that involve true malpractice from those that are brought by disappointed and frustrated patients.

Sue is a young woman with a long history of juvenile-onset diabetes. When Sue became legally blind, she sued her physician for malpractice. She charged her doctor with failing to fully disclose the risks of deviating from her prescribed diet and missing her ophthalmology exams. The doctor recalled discussing these issues with Sue on many occasions, but he could not document any particular discussions. Unable to defend himself against the charges, the doctor could be found guilty of medical malpractice.

Joe consents to a treatment that is ultimately unsuccessful. He charges his doctor with failing to provide adequate warning about the potential for a poor outcome. The judge must decide whether an overconfident doctor proceeded with a risky treatment without regard to the patient's wishes, or a discouraged patient is suffering from a case of sour grapes.

Regardless of the subtleties of state medical malpractice statutes, this much is clear: A patient who signs a consent form does not give up any right to sue a doctor for malpractice. A doctor who negligently performs a medical procedure is guilty of malpractice, regardless of the breadth of the patient's consent. A signed consent form only proves that the patient received information about, and approved, the procedure described on the form. Patients can never sign away their right to receive competent and appropriate medical care. (Medical malpractice is covered in depth in chapter 1.)

DISCLOSURE REQUIREMENTS OF MEDICAL SCREENING

The goal of medical screening is to detect potentially dangerous medical conditions before they become full-blown medical crises. Medical screening, just like any other medical treatment, test, or operation, cannot be performed without the patient's prior consent.

Advances in genetic research have spawned new concerns about informed consent and medical screening. Researchers can now use genetic screening tests to isolate many disease-causing genes. This new technology enables them to identify individuals who are likely to become afflicted with a particular disease in the future. Tests designed to detect genetic abnormalities are a novel type of medical screening. According to the Institute of Medicine's Committee on Assessing Genetic Risks, standard medical practice will include genetic testing based upon a single blood or tissue sample as early as the beginning of the next century.

Soon to enter the marketplace are genetic tests that can tell if a person is likely to get cancer. The tests, which will cost as little as $150, promise to identify an inherited predisposition to breast cancer, colon cancer, melanoma, thyroid cancer, and brain tumors. The tests analyze genes obtained from blood samples or swabbings from the inside of the patient's cheek.[45] In January 1996 a genetic test that could provide early warning of a high risk for breast or ovarian cancer became the first such test available outside cancer research centers.

A medical center in Tampa, Florida, has begun offering a test to predict the likelihood of developing Alzheimer's disease. The test is being given as part of a study into the Apo-E genes, which have been linked to the devastating and debilitating disease. A positive test result may indicate an enhanced risk of developing Alzheimer's disease—perhaps an increase of fifteen times the risk faced by the normal population. Thus far, researchers have not disclosed the test results to the subjects who have been tested.

Janet Walsh, the forty-year-old president of the Long Island Alzheimer's Foundation, is frustrated by her inability to learn whether her genetic composition destines her to the same fate that befell her father and maternal grandmother, both of whom had Alzheimer's. She wants to know whether she should make arrangements for her future care, read *Final Exit* and join the Hemlock Society (see page 175). In Walsh's opinion, she has a right to this information about her future. A 1995 study of people at risk of developing Alzheimer's found that 63 percent would opt to take a genetic test for the disease, if given the opportunity, even though there is no known cure.

The Florida researchers may soon start disclosing the results of the Alzheimer's test. They are establishing a clinic where genetic information can be disclosed in a supportive environment that makes appropriate counseling available. Also, new medical research shows that patients with one of the four variations of the Apo-E gene are less likely to respond to Tacrine, the only federally-approved drug for Alzheimer's disease. Other doctors pledge to continue to withhold the test results until there is a preventative treatment for Alzheimer's disease.

Interestingly, Apo-E testing also has proven effective in predicting treatable heart disease. Doctors involved in the treatment and research of heart disease routinely order Apo-E blood tests without intending to learn their patients' risk of developing Alzheimer's disease. Leaders at an October 1995 meeting sponsored by the Alzheimer's Association and the National Institute on Aging decided that doctors who used the Apo-E test for purposes other than predicting susceptibility to Alzheimer's disease were not obliged to inform their patients of the gene's connection to risk of Alzheimer's.

Results from a genetic test for Huntington's disease have been available to patients for years. Huntington's disease, like Alzheimer's disease, is severely disabling, can onset in late middle age, and is not currently preventable. There is, however, an important difference between the two tests. The Huntington's test in "predictive." A subject who gets a positive test result will develop Huntington's disease, unlike the Alzheimer's test, which merely reveals an increased risk of developing the disease. The majority of family members who may have the Huntington's disease gene have opted against learning whether they will get the disease; a minority have learned the results primarily to help them decide whether to have children.

Who should be responsible for consenting to genetic testing? Should parents have exclusive decision-making authority when it comes to testing their children for genetic "flaws," or does the government have a role to play?

The federal government has studied genetic testing to determine the extent to which the tests should be made available. The government's primary concerns are that scientists still do not fully understand the significance of mutated genes, and patients who learn about an increased risk of contracting a cancer that cannot be prevented will become depressed or suicidal. The federal government's Human Genome Project has learned in its survey of families where at least one person has an inherited genetic disease that most respondents strongly believed that parents should be allowed to have their children tested for diseases that are treatable, but that the government should prohibit testing for diseases that cannot be treated or prevented.

The government's finding was endorsed by the author of an article published in the September 1994 issue of the *Journal of the American Medical Association*.[46] In the article, Dr. Dorothy C. Wertz argues that genetic testing should be readily available only if the child stands to derive a direct medical benefit from the test results. While Dr. Wertz favors childhood testing for hypercholesterolemia (a cause of high cholesterol), which can be treated, she disapproves of testing for Alzheimer's disease, which remains untreatable. The obvious concern is that testing for untreatable medical conditions could unnecessarily damage a child's self-esteem or cause emotional distress.

Ann Fagan, together with her eleven- and thirteen-year-old daughters, decided to proceed with a genetic test that would reveal whether the children had inherited a gene that causes familia polyposis. Familia polyposis leads to colon cancer. Ms. Fagan had been diagnosed with familia polyposis when she was twenty-six years old, and eventually had her colon and rectum removed. Each of her daughters had a 50 percent chance of inheriting the defective gene.

The tests revealed that both girls had inherited the defective gene, and would eventually have to have their colons and rectums removed. Although Ms. Fagan recognized that many parents would not have chosen to have their children tested, she believed her family needed to know.[47]

One of the critical pieces of information that should be disclosed to a patient who is asked to consent to a screening procedure, genetic or otherwise, is the risk of an erroneous test result. Almost every medical screening technique occasionally yields incorrect results called false-positive and false-negative findings. A false-positive test result indicates a problem in the absence of any medical cause, and a false-negative test result shows no problem despite the presence of a medical abnormality. The consequences of a false-positive or false-negative result can range from merely inconvenient to dangerous, painful, or emotionally devastating.

Say you get a telephone call from your gynecologist. Your Pap smear came back positive. You are convinced you are dying of cervical cancer. When your hands stop shaking long enough to dial the telephone, you schedule a follow-up colposcopy. The invasive test is unpleasant, to say the least, and expensive. A few days later you get the call; the colposcopy was negative. The Pap smear falsely indicated that there was a problem (a false-positive result). You don't know whether to be extremely relieved or extremely annoyed.

A false-negative test result can be equally troubling. You finally go in for an electrocardiogram, and the test fails to detect an irregularity in your heartbeat. Instead of making appropriate changes in your behavior and eating habits, and starting a medication regimen, you go about your business as usual. You continue working at your high-stress job and eating your high-fat lunches. The delayed diagnosis and treatment of your cardiac condition could prove fatal.

Patients who suffer as a result of false-positive or false-negative test results sometimes have legal recourse. The burden of proving that the screening process had not been adequately explained beforehand, including the risk of inaccurate results, falls on the patient.

The problem of inadequate disclosure and medical screening is becoming somewhat more pressing as the pace of medical screening picks up. Possibly out of fear of a medical malpractice suit, physicians are prescribing screening tests with increasing frequency. A 1993 study reported in the *New England Journal of Medicine* found that family doctors are screening their patients more often than recommended by the U.S. Preventive Services Task Force.[48] Screening people at low risk for a disease may subject patients to unnecessary anxiety and put an additional drain on the nation's health care resources.

RIGHTS OF MINORS

At first blush, the law governing the rights of minors to give and withhold consent to proposed medical treatment is deceptively straightforward. However, many difficult issues lurk just beneath the surface.

In most states, minors under age fourteen are deemed incapable of giving informed consent to medical treatment.[49] Teenagers age fourteen and older who are found to be capable of understanding the treatment, as well as its risks, benefits, and alternatives, are authorized to obtain medical services without a parent's approval. Teenagers who fall into this category are frequently referred to as "mature minors." Adolescents serving in the armed forces can also legally consent to their own treatment, as can adolescents living away from home who manage their own financial affairs.[50]

Certain types of medical treatments do not require parental consent, regardless of the minor's status. These exceptions are spelled out in state medical emancipation statutes. Typically, minors are allowed to consent to pregnancy care, contraceptive services, treatment for sexually transmitted diseases, and alcohol and other drug abuse treatment without parental involvement. Some states also permit minors to consent to mental health treatment.[51]

Where the child is not authorized to consent to the proposed treatment, doctors generally look to parents and legal guardians to consent to medical procedures on behalf of their children. In cases involving divorce, consent is required from the custodial parent. Stepparents cannot usually give consent, and foster parents may be authorized to consent, depending on the state.

Parents and legal guardians who are asked to consent to a medical procedure on a minor's behalf are held accountable to the state. The state has the authority to ensure that treatment decisions made by parents are, in fact, in the best interests of their children. Parents who refuse on religious grounds to consent to medical procedures on their children's behalf may have their decision overridden by a judge.

Take, for example, Lee Lor, a fifteen-year-old Hmong girl whose family comes from the mountains of Southeast Asia. Hmongs only believe in the use of herbal remedies to treat illness. Lee Lor was a resident of California when she was diagnosed with cancer.

Lee Lor's parents refused to allow their daughter to be taken to the hospital for chemotherapy. The California Department of Social Services asked a judge to intervene, and a court order was issued authorizing the police to forcibly remove the young girl from her home.[52]

The conflict between the state's interest in preserving life and in the family's right to practice their religion could not have been more stark. According to doctors, Lee Lor stood only a 10 percent chance of surviving without chemotherapy. If she started immediate chemotherapy treatments, she had an 80 percent chance of survival.

After a week of chemotherapy, Lee Lor returned home for a visit. Not surprisingly, she disappeared. Her family filed a missing person report but refused to provide police with Lee Lor's picture or the telephone numbers of friends and family. The court order authorizing treatment became moot.

The right of a minor to withhold consent to treatment became a hot topic of debate both within and outside the health care industry on October 26, 1994, when Billy Best, a sixteen-year-old teenager diagnosed with a curable form of lymphatic cancer, ran away from home to avoid additional chemotherapy treatments. He left behind a note: "The reason I left is because I could not stand going to the hospital every week. I feel like the medicine is killing me instead of helping me." Suddenly the public spotlight was turned on the rights of minors to withhold consent to medical care.[53]

Once again, the dilemma was clear: Was Billy, a teenager, capable of making short-term sacrifices for long-term health benefits, or did his expectation of immediate gratification render him incapable of making a rational treatment decision? Should any teenager who has the typical adolescent concerns about physical appearance be expected to willingly undergo a treatment that causes hair loss and weight gain?

In the opinion of Dr. Arthur Caplan, the director of the Center for Bioethics at the University of Pennsylvania, teenagers should have the right to withhold consent to treatment. Just as the law gives "mature minors" who can understand the consequences of their decisions the right to consent to treatment, Dr. Caplan argues, mature minors should have the right to make informed decisions to *withhold* consent. Many doctors also find that, as a practical matter, adolescents who are given control over their treatment decisions are more likely to comply with recommended treatments.

When Billy voluntarily returned home in November 1994, his parents called a press conference. They announced that the chemotherapy treatments would be discontinued, and that the choice of future treatments would be left to Billy. (Billy was also approached by book publishers and producers of tabloid television shows with generous offers to buy his story.) Mrs. Best expressed regret that she had not insisted that Billy join a support group. (Sources of information about support groups are included in appendix 7.)

Nonconsensual drug testing of minors raises similar concerns. A thirteen-year-old is brought to the pediatrician's office by his mother for a general checkup. At one point in the examination, the pediatrician shines a flashlight into the youth's nasal passages. What she sees leads her to suspect that her patient has been snorting cocaine on a regular basis for an extended period of time. Can the doctor test the patient for drug use without his consent?

This question has divided the medical community. The official position of the American Academy of Pediatrics (AAP) is that involuntary drug tests should not be conducted on competent older adolescents without the informed consent of the patient, even if the testing is requested by the patient's parents. Medical professionals within and outside the AAP disagree.

There is no easy answer. Physicians resolve this difficult issue by carefully weighing the adolescent's right to privacy and confidentiality against the interests of the child's parents and the state in protecting the adolescent's well-being. Those who oppose the AAP guidelines argue that waiver of consent is appropriate when drug abuse is suspected. A drug-abusing adolescent may not be competent to make decisions about his or her care, and the adolescent may face serious and irreparable harm if drug use is allowed to continue undetected and untreated.

The American Academy of Child and Adolescent Psychiatry (AACAP) disagrees with the AAP guidelines. A 1991 policy statement issued by the AACAP sets forth the organization's position: "Confidentiality is not unconditional when the child's mental status is severely impaired or when the adolescent is judged to be in a life-threatening situation. It may be appropriate, however, to obtain informed consent for testing from the parents when the minor patient exhibits poor judgment, cannot make a positive treatment alliance, is dangerous to himself or herself, or to others, does not show concern for his or her condition, and/or refuses help."[54]

DISCLOSURE AND ABORTION RIGHTS

Few would dispute that abortion is one of the most divisive issues of the day. Advocates on both sides of the fence hold strong convictions about when life begins, the extent of a woman's right to privacy, and the state's interest in preserving life. A relatively new issue in the abortion debate is the role of informed consent.

A number of states have passed informed consent laws that apply specifically to women seeking abortions. These laws often share similar provisions. They generally require physicians to describe to the woman, at least twenty-four hours before the abortion is performed, the nature of the abortion procedure, including risks and alternatives, the probable gestational age of the fetus, and the medical risks of carrying the pregnancy to term. Usually printed material must also be made available to the pregnant woman. Such literature describes the physical characteristics of the embryo or fetus, lists agencies that provide abortion alternatives and assistance, and explains the father's support obligations.

Those who favor the mandatory informed consent laws use the slogan of abortion rights advocates to make their point. They argue that abortion rights advocates are not being consistent when they urge free choice for women yet oppose informed consent legislation. How, the argument goes, can a woman freely choose to continue or terminate a pregnancy if she does not have access to all of the relevant information regarding that choice?

Public opinion polls have found that people who favor legalized abortion do not necessarily oppose state mandatory informed consent legislation. A 1990 Wirthlin Group poll, for example, found that 84 percent of men and 89 percent of women surveyed would support legislation "requiring women to receive information about fetal development and alternatives to abortion before going ahead with the procedure."

The American Medical Association, the American College of Obstetricians and Gynecologists, abortion rights groups, and others counter that mandatory informed consent laws are drafted to discourage abortions. The laws require doctors to make biased presentations of medical information to their patients, in particular by discussing the fetus's gestational development. They also compel physicians to discuss with their pregnant patients such matters as child support and welfare eligibility, which fall outside their realm of expertise.

Opponents of the mandatory informed consent laws have proposed alternative informed consent requirements. Under these alternative proposals, doctors would be required to explain to their patients the nature and consequences of the abortion procedure. The doctors would only be responsible for providing their pregnant patients with enough information to enable those patients to make a knowledgeable decision about whether to proceed with the abortion. The doctors would not have to raise any extraneous matters that might influence the patient's decision one way or the other.

The U.S. Supreme Court's position on informed consent legislation has changed dramatically over the last decade. In 1986 the court struck down a state's informed consent statute because it required doctors to disclose fetal development information to the patient. The Court held that such information "is not medical information that is always relevant to a woman's decision, and it may serve only to confuse and punish her and to heighten her anxiety, contrary to accepted medical practice."[55] The statutory requirement mandating the disclosure of certain facts was found to violate patients' rights of privacy.

A few years later, on June 29, 1992, the Supreme Court in *Planned Parenthood v. Casey* upheld several consent provisions of Pennsylvania's abortion law.[56] Under the Pennsylvania law, doctors are required to inform women of the fetus's probable gestational age and advise their patients of their right to view material about fetal development published by the state health department. The physician or other counselor must also inform the patient about state programs that provide medical assistance benefits if the fetus is carried to term, and the father's legal responsibility to provide support. Twenty-four hours must pass between the giving of the mandated information and the abortion. In the case of a minor, at least one parent must be present during these discussions and give consent unless a judge rules otherwise.

The right to have an abortion, though guaranteed by the U.S. Constitution, is regulated by state, not federal, law. Accordingly, mandatory consent laws are a creation of state, not federal, legislators.

The Supreme Court's newfound tolerance for mandatory disclosure provisions is best understood in the context of abortion rights decisions generally.

Traditionally, abortion rights decisions were grounded on a constitutional right of privacy. Any attempt to intrude on the confidentiality of the patient-physician relationship was struck down as a violation of a woman's privacy interests.

The landmark abortion rights decisions of *Roe v. Wade* and *Doe v. Bolton*, for example, were both premised on the constitutional right of privacy. In each decision, the court recognized the importance of protecting private doctor-patient communications from undue governmental influence. Women were found to be free to seek the advice and assistance of their physicians without interference from the government.[57]

A growing number of Supreme Court justices now characterize the right to elect abortion as only a "liberty interest." Characterizing the right to an abortion as a liberty interest permits additional government regulation of abortion decisions.[58]

ECONOMIC INFORMED CONSENT

As America's health care resources have become increasingly strained, there has been talk of changing the scope of informed consent. Should doctors take the cost of alternative medical procedures into account when deciding what treatment options to discuss with their patients?

Take Linda's situation, for example. Linda was diagnosed with cancer. Her doctors agreed that she could be treated in one of three ways. She could undergo chemotherapy, radiation therapy, or an expensive new experimental drug treatment program. Linda's insurance covered only chemotherapy and radiation; experimental treatments were excluded. Since Linda had been too sick to work, she had depleted her savings and could not afford the $10,000 annual cost of the experimental drug. Is Linda's doctor obligated to discuss the experimental treatment with Linda, knowing that she cannot afford the treatment?

The patient's right of self-determination compels disclosure of all alternative medical treatments, even if the patient cannot afford them. Patients, not their doctors, should decide whether a treatment alternative is worth financial ruin. Perhaps Linda could borrow the money to pay for the experimental drugs, or appeal her insurer's denial of coverage, or qualify for some type of public assistance or charitable help.

Furthermore, patients are entitled to know about every treatment option, affordable or otherwise, because they pay their doctors for that information. Patients and doctors have a contractual relationship. Under this implied contract, the doctor is obligated to explore every available treatment alternative, and the patient is obligated to pay the doctor's fee. A doctor who learns about a treatment alternative on the patient's dime owes that patient full disclosure.

Finally, the doctor is the patient's fiduciary. As a fiduciary, the doctor is obligated to act on the patient's behalf in the patient's best interest. Disclosure of prohibitively expensive treatment options advances the patient's interests in improving the likelihood of finding an effective treatment or cure.

On the other side of the coin are medical ethicists who argue that patients give their implied consent to forgo certain costly medical procedures when they purchase less comprehensive health insurance or forgo insurance entirely. Under this theory, underinsured patients effectively consent in advance to the withholding of treatments with questionable cost effectiveness. A patient whose insurance does not cover costly experimental medical treatments, for example, may be found to have waived her right to receive information about the availability of treatments that have no history of success.

The issue of economic informed consent recently arose in the context of neonatal care, as illustrated by the controversy that swirled around Ryan Nguyen. Ryan was born on October 27, 1994, six weeks before his due date, asphyxiated and with barely a heartbeat. At two months of age he exhibited multiple medical problems including irreversible kidney failure, bowel obstructions, and moderate to severe brain damage. The cost of treating Ryan averaged $2,000 a day.

The neonatologists in the hospital where Ryan was born suggested to Ryan's parents that they consent to the termination of the dialysis treatments and let Ryan die. The parents refused to give their consent and hired an attorney. The attorney accused the doctors of deciding to allow Ryan to die because the parents could not afford the cost of caring for their son. The doctors denied the charges.

This case raises the difficult question of whether patients and their representatives should be given the opportunity to consent to all modes of treatment, even costly care that offers only a remote chance of saving life. This question will be left for another day. On December 13, 1994, doctors at a medical center in Portland, Oregon, agreed to continue treating Ryan. On March 6, 1995, little Ryan was discharged home.

While still shocking, the idea of economic consent may eventually gain greater acceptance. With many Americans unable to afford the most basic care, politicians and the public have been forced to revisit health care rationing. Health care rationing denies certain individuals access to needed medical services under specified circumstances. If health care rationing becomes a reality, economic informed consent may not be far behind.

RESOURCES

The National Women's Health Network (see page 37)

> **People Against Cancer**
> P. O. Box 10
> Otho, Iowa
> 515-972-4444
>
> *People Against Cancer is an advocacy organization that is skeptical of traditional clinical trials and standard cancer therapies.*

THREE

Your Rights of
Health Care Privacy

Perhaps no aspect of your life is more personal than your health care records. These records often do more than merely document your medical treatments and diagnoses. They can include information about your sexual habits, drug use, lifestyle, work environment, prior pregnancies, abortions, and your parents' causes of death. Your health care records can even include information about your income, education, and living arrangements.

The disclosure of health information can have widespread consequences as the following three examples, all drawn from recent history, demonstrate. When employees of the Princeton Medical Center got wind of the fact that a popular surgeon had tested positive for the AIDS virus, the surgeon's career ended. A student of the University of Cincinnati who charged two university employees with sexual harassment was humiliated when medical records documenting her sexual history were introduced into evidence. A New York congresswoman was disgraced when hospital records disclosing her suicide attempt were faxed to the media.

Despite the high stakes involved, the confidentiality of personal medical records has been left virtually unregulated. At present, no federal law specifically protects the privacy of medical records by regulating when medical records may be disclosed, and to whom. Greater national privacy protection is afforded banking records, library records, and video rental lists.

This chapter opens with a brief summary of the legal bases of informational privacy. The sections that follow discuss waiving your right to informational privacy, the record-keeping role of the Medical Information Bureau, privacy of medical records in the computer age, privacy concerns about medical testing, and adolescent health care privacy. The chapter concludes with a list of sources of additional information.

LEGAL BASES OF INFORMATIONAL PRIVACY

The Federal Privacy Act of 1974 is as close as the federal government has come to protecting the privacy of medical records on a national level. The Act protects citizens from the governmental disclosure of confidential information. Only medical records within the custody of the federal government fall under the purview of the law. Records retained by private medical institutions not under contract with the federal government are not subject to the privacy act.

The exclusion of private medical providers is not the only shortcoming of the Federal Privacy Act. The enforcement provisions of the act also leave something to be desired.

Remedies only become available under the privacy act *after* a patient's privacy has already been breached. Unfortunately, once the cat is out of the bag there may be no getting that cat back into the bag. The harm that flows from a broken confidence can, in other words, be irreparable.[59]

Other relevant federal legislation includes the Americans with Disabilities Act (ADA). The ADA applies to employers with fifteen or more workers (or smaller companies, depending on state law). Under the ADA, covered employers are only permitted to ask prospective employees for medical information after the employer has made a job offer, and only if the employer requests the same information from all other applicants. Medical information received from the employee can legally be used by the employer to withdraw a job offer only if the information establishes that the applicant is unable to perform the job. The employer cannot rely on the medical information to withdraw a job offer because the employer fears that the applicant poses an insurance risk, or if the applicant with the disability could perform the job with "reasonable accommodation." Federal regulations protect the confidentiality of records of patients who are treated for drug or alcohol dependency at federally funded facilities.

At the end of 1995, bipartisan support was growing for a new Medical Records Confidentiality Act. The bill would create a federal right to inspect, copy, and correct inaccurate personal records; prohibit health care providers from releasing data without patient consent or condition treatment on receiving that consent; and encourage the elimination of patient identifying information to protect the confidentiality of medical data that is legitimately exchanged. While civil libertarians and patients' rights advocates would like to see enhanced privacy protections, representatives of organized business generally support the bill.

States are, to say the least, inconsistent in the privacy protection they afford medical records. Only twenty-eight states offer any medical privacy rights. In some jurisdictions, the privacy of only select medical records is protected. While the records of patients afflicted with sexually transmitted diseases and acquired immunodeficiency syndrome (AIDS) may be protected, patients with other communicable diseases, such as tuberculosis, may receive little or no protection. No state law, however, can protect the confidentiality of data transmitted across state lines.

The Pennsylvania AIDS confidentiality law was the subject of a lawsuit brought by an obstetrician/gynecologist against the medical center that had employed him. The doctor had gone for a voluntary AIDS test after he was cut while delivering a baby. When the test came back positive, the doctor promptly resigned from the hospital. Shortly after the doctor submitted his resignation, the hospital asked the county court for permission to publicize the doctor's positive test result. The judge consented to the disclosure based on a finding of a "compelling need." The court accepted the argument of the hospital's attorneys that disclosure was appropriate given the possibility that the doctor exposed his patients to HIV infection.[60]

The doctor appealed on the ground that there had been no compelling need to disclose the results of his AIDS test. He argued that disclosure was unwarranted in the absence of evidence that he had actually exposed any patients to the virus. He further argued that to order disclosure under the circumstances would set bad public policy. Other physicians who suspected that they might be infected with HIV might fear the consequences of undergoing voluntary testing. The result could be a more rapid spread of the AIDS epidemic. The physician lost the appeal.[61]

AIDS confidentiality laws vary from state to state. Some jurisdictions require the individual's prior consent to disclosure of the test results. Others allow disclosure of test results to organ banks, blood banks, state health agencies, and the individual's personal physician without the individual's consent. Where no legislation applies specifically to AIDS, the general state statute on medical records applies.

Federal legislation has been proposed to protect the privacy of people who suffer from stigmatizing medical conditions. The goal of the legislation would be to encourage patients with such conditions to receive the testing, counseling, and treatment they require. The legislation would permit disclosure of the medical records to specified individuals and agencies, including spouses, sexual contacts, blood, organ, semen, and breast milk banks, certain health care workers, and public health officers. The future of the legislation remains uncertain.

Many state laws allow medical providers to release a patient's medical records only with the patient's consent. As a practical matter, the effectiveness of this statutory protection is limited. Patients routinely knowingly and unknowingly waive their right of privacy. When you apply for a job, insurance, or a loan, you often sign a medical release as part of the application. By signing the release, you consent to the disclosure of your personal medical records. (Medical releases are covered in greater depth in the following section.)

Federal and state statutes are not the only sources of protection of informational privacy. Additional safeguards can be found in both the federal and state constitutions.

The U.S. Supreme Court first articulated the federal constitutional right to privacy in a case involving government data banks.[62] The case involved a government database of lawful users of abusable drugs. The Court was asked to decide how much security was enough security to prevent any constitutional harm to the persons listed in the data bank. The Court held that stringent security measures were required to protect the privacy of sensitive medical information.[63]

The constitutional right to informational privacy was revisited by a federal appeals court three years later. The appellate court said that five factors should be balanced in determining the adequacy of privacy protections of medical records:

1. The type of health record and information at issue
2. The potential for harm from any unauthorized disclosure
3. The manner in which the record was generated
4. The adequacy of safeguards to prevent nonconsensual disclosure
5. The degree of need for access.

The adequacy of the privacy protections must be evaluated on a case-by-case basis.[64]

More recently a unanimous federal appeals court found that the constitutional right to privacy protects people infected with the AIDS virus from exposure by public agencies. The finding was made in a case involving a Delta Airlines employee who claimed that co-workers were able to figure out he had the AIDS virus after the New York City Human Rights Commission issued a press release concerning his job discrimination claim. Although the press release did not identify the man by name, it provided sufficient information to make him identifiable by others.[65]

Judicial interpretations of the constitutional right of privacy only apply to governmental agencies; the U.S. Constitution does not reach private entities. State constitutional protections of informational privacy also apply primarily to governmental agencies. Only in limited cases have the strictures been applied to private parties.[66]

The venerable doctor-patient privilege provides an additional source of protection against the wrongful disclosure of personal medical information. The origin of this privilege can be traced back to the Hippocratic oath: "Whatsoever I shall see or hear in the course of my profession ... if it be what should not be published abroad, I will never divulge, holding such things to be holy secrets." Doctors are supposed to exercise discretion in divulging the confidences of their patients.

The doctor-patient privilege is legally recognized in all fifty states. Physicians and psychotherapists cannot be compelled to disclose patient records or testify about a patient in a judicial proceeding. This privilege, however, only goes so far. Although doctors are legally prohibited from spilling the beans on the witness stand, they are only morally prohibited from letting their lips flap outside the courtroom. Furthermore, the privilege has rarely been extended to unauthorized disclosures made by non-physicians in the health care industry, such as loose-lipped researchers, laboratory technicians, and nurses' aides, and has been found to disappear when the public's well-being is at stake. Doctors must report cases of venereal disease to the Centers for Disease Control, privilege or no privilege.

In federal court, the situation is different. Although the federal courts have long respected a physician-patient privilege, they have split on the issue of a psychotherapist-patient privilege. In October 1995 the U.S. Supreme Court agreed to decide whether communications between mental health workers and their patients may not be ordered disclosed in court.

WAIVING YOUR PRIVACY PROTECTIONS

Unbeknownst to you, you may routinely be relinquishing what little control you have over the privacy of your health records.

When you apply for insurance, employment, or credit, do you read all of the small print on the application? Do you know whether you are giving the insurer, employer, or credit agency access to information about your health?

When you sign a medical release as part of an application, you may be opening the window to your personal life wider than you'd like. A typical medical authorization reads as follows:

> *To all physicians, surgeons and other medical practitioners, all hospitals, clinics and other health care delivery facilities, all insurance carriers, insurance data service organizations and health maintenance organizations, who may have records or evidence relating to my physical or mental condition, I hereby authorize release and delivery of any and all information, records and documents, confidential or otherwise, with respect to my health and health history that you, or any of you, now have or hereafter obtain.*

The expansiveness of this release is self-evident. Such a form, once signed, can be copied and used over and over, at any time, and for any purpose.

Before rushing to sign such an all-inclusive authorization, consider respectfully requesting permission to modify the authorization. Assure whoever is asking you to sign the form that the changes you would like to make will not impede his or her ability to obtain information about you. The changes will affect only the ability of other people to use the form at other times for other purposes.

If you get permission to modify the form, here are some changes you might want to make:

➤ Write in the name of the particular hospital, clinic, or physician that is being asked to release information.

➤ Identify the specific medical information being sought, either by the nature of the illness or injury or the time period. For example, limit the request to records pertaining to your broken leg or records dated January through April, 1995.

➤ Include a clause that the medical records obtained under the release can only be used for certain purposes, such as a particular application for insurance or employment.

You may also want to have a conversation with the intended recipient of the authorization, typically your doctor. Ask the provider to keep to a minimum the medical information that is disclosed under the authorization. Many doctors are quick to copy and distribute a patient's entire medical record rather than take the time to search the record for the particular information that is the subject of the authorization. Let your doctor know that you do not consent to the disclosure of your entire medical file.

The only time you should probably not even ask to modify the medical release is if you are being asked to sign the form by a self-insured employer. Such a request might put your job at risk. Self-insured companies use corporate funds to cover their workers' medical expenses. About 250 Fortune 500 companies are self-insured. Self-insured employers have a direct financial interest in having unlimited access to information about their employees' medical conditions.

As a general matter, employees of self-insured companies have a tougher time maintaining their health care privacy. Each time they file a claim for coverage of a medical expense, they disclose to their employer something else about their medical condition and personal life.

If you work for a self-insured employer, you may want to find out who processes the insurance claims. Who within the company has access to the insurance records? Your benefits officer at work should be able to provide you with this information.

This information about your company's claims-processing policies, while interesting, will not be of much practical use. Self-insured employers are usually exempt from state regulations that govern the privacy of medical records maintained by independent insurance companies. You may, however, draw comfort from the knowledge that only one or two corporate employees have access to your claims information.

Although employers who purchase coverage for their workers from private insurers do not have the same direct access to claims information as self-insured employers, they usually keep in close touch with their insurers. In many cases, the private insurance carriers openly convey to the employers a willingness to share claims information concerning employees. The insurers know who pays the insurance premiums—your employer, not you.

What's so bad, you might wonder, about your employer finding out that you had gallstones removed last year or were diagnosed with an ulcer the year before?

Unfortunately, the disclosure of medical information *can* yield devastating results. The wrong piece of medical information whispered in the ears of the wrong employer can mean the loss of a job. Half of the Fortune 500 companies that responded to a 1989 poll conceded that they use health information to make employment-related decisions. Of those, 19 percent reported that they did not inform the employee of such use.[67] Another study reported by the Office of Technology Assessment found that many companies will not hire applicants who have a preexisting medical condition.[68]

New concerns are being raised as the use of company doctors increases. Sometimes the company doctor is a doctor who offers employees inexpensive preventive care as part of an employer's "wellness program." These company doctors screen employees for heart disease or breast cancer, or test for high cholesterol or blood pressure. Other company doctors are more like employer-run health maintenance organizations, offering a broader selection of medical services.

A visit to a company doctor can open the door to a host of problems. What if you are diagnosed with a condition that will be costly to treat? According to a spokesperson from the American Civil Liberties Union, you risk losing your coverage and/or your job.

The consequences of a confidentiality breach can also be devastating. In one case, employees experienced workplace problems after news of their HIV-positive status leaked out of the company doctor's office. In another case, a supervisor pressured a manager to leave on disability after rumors of the manager's medical problems became common knowledge within the company.

Many experts in medical privacy recommend approaching company doctors with caution. Although these experts feel comfortable recommending the use of a company doctor for flu shots and cancer screenings (especially for procrastinators who would otherwise go without the preventive tests), most warn employees against going to a company doctor for much else.

Employees are warned against going to a company doctor for a hearing test if the test might reveal a more-than-mild hearing problem; for allergy shots, because the employer might decide the worker should not perform tasks that might trigger an allergic reaction (a decision better left to the worker and his or her personal physician); for blood pressure or cholesterol testing, since the results could flag the employee as an insurance risk; or for urinalysis, a test that reveals a wealth of information about private matters. Most importantly, workers are advised against going to a company doctor for genetic screening or HIV testing. The risk of discrimination based on these test results is too substantial.

You may be surprised to learn that you disclose personal information about your health every day, without ever putting a pen to a medical authorization form or visiting the company doctor. When you pay for your drug store purchases with a credit card, for example, you create a record of your dry skin condition, need for extra fiber, or method of birth control. When you call that toll-free customer service number on your tube of toothpaste, your name joins a list of people with sensitive teeth, discolored teeth, or plaque-ridden teeth. When you accept a free blood pressure check at your local drugstore, you create a record that can be sold to drug manufacturers for marketing purposes. When you subscribe to a newsletter about health and fitness, return a rebate coupon for diet pills, or buy vitamins through the mail, your name (and the mailing list on which it appears) may be destined for the desk of the marketing executive who is willing to pay the right price for it.

Information about our use of prescription drugs is a particularly hot commodity. Prescription information is routinely released by doctors and pharmacists to data collectors. These data collectors sell the information to pharmaceutical companies for marketing purposes.

Those who participate in this practice argue that there is no threat to patient privacy because the pharmaceutical companies are only interested in statistical information about drug use and outcomes. They are not interested in identifying the drug users themselves. In fact, the patient's name is often deleted when the statistical information is compiled.[69]

Opponents respond that the deletion of the user's name does not provide adequate privacy protection. Deleted information can always be restored.

Computerized drug-tracking systems can now identify patients and the doctors who prescribe drugs to them. More and more states are using these systems to reduce illegal drug trafficking. Although the U.S. Drug Enforcement Administration reports that drug crimes have been reduced in the eleven states with drug-tracking systems, many fear that outside monitoring of doctors' prescribing practices violates the privacy of the doctor-patient relationship. There is also concern that doctors, knowing they are being watched, will be intimidated into changing their prescribing practices to the detriment of their patients.

Police in one Ohio town went even further. They began collecting drug use data from local pharmacies in an effort to control drug crimes. Residents challenged the program under state laws that limit public access to pharmaceutical records. The program was upheld in court based on a finding that the state laws did not apply to controlled substances, and the loss of privacy was justified by the increased protection against drug crimes.[70]

In recognition of patient vulnerability to breaches of confidentiality with respect to the use of prescription drugs, federal legislators have made attempts to regulate on a national level the disclosure of pharmacy records. The proposed Prescription Drug Records Privacy Protection Act was one such attempt. This bill, which was introduced to Congress in 1992, made the unauthorized disclosure of pharmacy records punishable by law. As of yet, Congress has not taken action on any such legislation.

Unless and until laws are passed protecting our right to informational privacy, you must assume responsibility for protecting information about your health from informational pirates. Here are some steps you can take to keep your use of prescription drugs, and other health care matters, private.

➤ Request that your name be removed from many national mailing lists. To make such a request, send your complete name, address, and zip code to

Direct Marketing Association, Mail Preference Service, P.O. Box 9008, Farmingdale, New York 11735-9008. For more information, call 212-768-7277.

➤ Be careful about when and to whom you disclose personal information. Think twice before you complete that questionnaire you received in the mail asking you about the products you use. No one needs to know how often you take decongestants, your antacid of choice, and whether you subscribe to any health magazines.

➤ When you return a warranty card on a new appliance, such as an electric shaver or plaque remover, include only your name, address, and telephone number. Information about your income, marital status, and buying habits are solicited solely for marketing purposes. You do not have to provide this information (and may not even be required to return the card) to get the benefit of the warranty.

➤ Beware of inadvertent disclosures of personal medical information. Remember that you are not anonymous when you make a telephone call. Many businesses now use caller ID. Caller ID gives the recipient of the call the caller's telephone number. Your telephone number is the key to your name and address, which can be located in a reverse telephone book or other more sophisticated identification technique.

➤ Recognize that you create a record of your purchases every time you use your credit card. Anyone who has ever scrutinized the contents of another person's supermarket shopping cart knows how much you can learn about another person from his or her purchases. Instead of whipping out a credit card to make purchases that you would just as soon keep private, use cash.

➤ Review your own medical records. Make sure the information in your medical file is accurate. To get a copy of your medical file, send a letter of request to every doctor, hospital, and clinic that has treated you. If the provider refuses to send you a copy of your records, make sure you get that refusal in writing. Your right to review your medical records may be protected by state law. Over thirty states have such laws in place.

Governor Pataki of New York recently stripped patients of an additional aspect of their privacy. Now patients who voluntarily enter state-run mental hospitals in New York relinquish the privacy of their criminal records. Hospitals have access to a computerized list of their patients' outstanding warrants, arrests, and convictions—information that had previously been available only to law enforcement agencies. Patient rights advocates fear that providers will use a patient's criminal history to justify inappropriate treatment, and that the disclosure of this information will discourage patients from seeking treatment. The governor has also called for a law empowering judges to order HIV tests for criminal suspects on the request of the victims.

MEDICAL RECORDS, PRIVACY, AND THE MEDICAL INFORMATION BUREAU

Most people would agree that insurance companies should have special rights of access to private medical information. After all, when you get sick, the insurance company gets stuck paying your bill. But what restrictions, if any, should limit your insurer's ability to *disseminate* private medical information about you?

The primary threat to the confidentiality of medical information you provide to your insurer is posed by the Medical Information Bureau (MIB). The MIB is the health data clearinghouse for insurers.

Here's how the MIB works. You disclose medical information to the Good Hands Insurance Company when you apply for coverage. Good Hands forwards this information to the MIB. Two years later, you apply for coverage with State Barn Insurance Company. State Barn reviews your MIB record and becomes privy to the information you had previously disclosed to Good Hands.

MIB maintains a database of underwriting information. Underwriting information is information that bears on the risk an insured person poses to an insurer. Sedentary lifestyles, above-average weights, and higher-than-normal blood pressures are of infinite interest to underwriters.

MIB was established to discourage fraud among insurance applicants. The idea was to maintain a record of previously disclosed information about insurability so that applicants would have a tougher time omitting or concealing relevant information about themselves on subsequent applications for insurance coverage.

If you have ever applied for life insurance, you may have your own MIB file. About 680 life insurance companies report to the MIB. Approximately one out of every seven Americans has an MIB record.

Insurance companies that belong to the MIB send a coded report to the MIB whenever an applicant reports on an application for coverage "a condition significant to health or longevity." The most commonly reported conditions include EKG readings, X-rays, height, weight, and blood pressure signs. Non-medical information that might affect insurability, such as driving records and participation in hazardous sports, is also reported.

When Tom applied for insurance (life, health, or disability), he received an MIB notice. The notice advised him that the insurance company might make a report to the MIB, and might exchange the report with other member insurance companies. The notice further advised Tom how he could access and correct his MIB record.

As part of the application process, Tom signed an MIB Statement of Authorization. The authorization gave the insurer permission to obtain Tom's MIB report. (The MIB notice and authorization are reprinted in appendix 8.)

Tom, in a previous insurance application, had disclosed a family history of heart disease. The insurer had reported this information to the MIB as "a condition significant to health or longevity." Unfortunately for Tom, information about his passion for bungee jumping, record of speeding tickets, and childhood problem with obesity also made its way into his MIB record.

Insurers are allowed to use the MIB report only to detect fraud. The law prohibits insurance companies from making coverage decisions based on an MIB report.[71] All underwriting decisions must be based on information provided by the applicant, medical professionals, hospitals, laboratories, and other health care facilities.

The new insurer, upon receiving Tom's MIB report, compared the MIB report and Tom's current insurance application for inconsistencies. It investigated the discrepancies. When it did not find any fraud, the insurer issued Tom a policy.

As of October 1995, insurance applicants have a right to know whether their insurance application has been denied, or their premiums raised, as a result of their MIB record. Under the new rules, which resulted from an agreement entered into between the Federal Trade Commission and the private MIB organization, the MIB must disclose that information obtained from the MIB was used to reject an insurance application or raise premiums.

You cannot, and should not, assume that the information in your MIB report is accurate. For example, your MIB report might include a notation about a back condition because you made a passing comment to the insurance agent that your boss gave you "a pain in the neck." You must take responsibility for ensuring the accuracy of your MIB record.

There are many convoluted ways in which incorrect information finds its way into an MIB report. Say a patient reports fatigue after twenty minutes of exertion; his MIB file might indicate fatigue after two minutes of exertion due to a typographical error. A patient tells her doctor that she has been feeling "stressed out" lately; her MIB report might indicate an anxiety disorder. A pregnant woman who asks her obstetrician about the effect of marijuana use on fetal development might be surprised to find a notation in her MIB file indicating a history of drug use.

The MIB does not independently verify the information it includes in its records. Investigations into the accuracy of the information only follows a consumer's formal challenge to the accuracy of his or her MIB file. You can find out if there is a MIB file on you and its accuracy by contacting the Medical Information Bureau at the address and number that appears in the resource section at the end of this chapter.[72]

When you contact the MIB, you will be asked to complete a one-page request form. MIB promises to disclose or correct your record within thirty business days. MIB claims that about 800 of the approximately 50,000 people who request copies of their MIB record each year request corrections.

Unfortunately, errors on an MIB record can have a ripple effect. Although the error itself can be easily corrected, your MIB file may already have been released to several other insurance companies by the time the correction is made. The effects of the error can plague you for months or even years.

MEDICAL RECORDS, PRIVACY, AND COMPUTERS

Invasions of our informational privacy, though common, are still disturbing. A 1993 Harris-Equifax poll found 80 percent of respondents concerned about the privacy of their health records. About the same percentage of respondents felt that they had lost control over the dissemination and use of personal information about them.[73] As medical technology advances, and our use of computers becomes more sophisticated, the threat to the privacy of our medical information is only likely to increase.

Take, for example, the new privacy risks associated with advanced genetic technology. Scientists now store genetic information in DNA data banks. Despite the extremely personal nature of this genetic information, DNA data banks are barely subject to privacy controls. The laboratory can freely allow access to the stored information without even seeking the permission of the individuals whose DNA samples are on deposit.[74]

Similarly, the capacity of personal computer (PC) systems is being stretched to the limit as more and more information is being maintained about the growing number of people exposed to the Human Immunodeficiency Virus (HIV) and actual cases of Acquired Immunodeficiency Syndrome (AIDS). Public health agencies, state governments, and armed services branches all track cases of AIDS and HIV infection. The inadequacy of PC systems to maintain the growing numbers HIV- and AIDS-related records puts the confidentiality of these records at risk.

Although doctors and hospitals have been using computers for years to store information about payment and insurance coverage, computers are now storing substantive information about patients and every aspect of their medical history to an unprecedented extent. Can the confidentiality of personal health data be maintained as the health industry enters the computer age?

As long as computers store and transmit data electronically, there is a potential for abuse. Electronic data can be illicitly intercepted and examined by unauthorized entities at remote locations. It has happened before.

Employees of the Internal Revenue Service were once caught illegally searching the computerized tax records of celebrities. Private investigators hired by adopted children looking for their biological parents, or estranged spouses looking for evidence of deceit, have been known to rely on computerized information for breakthroughs.

Perhaps the most insidious aspect of computer security breaches is that they are invisible. An individual can be baffled by a series of rejections for employment, insurance, credit, and housing, only to learn that some incriminating medical information has been uncovered and widely disseminated.

Groups and individuals who may be interested in your medical records include employers, government agencies, credit bureaus, insurers, educational institutions, and the media. Drug manufacturers, marketing companies, medical suppliers, private investigators, lawyers, and your sworn enemies may also have reasons to seek access to information about your health. Even in the health care setting, numerous non-physician health care workers, among them nutritionists, therapists, social workers, pharmacists, medical students, and technicians, may want to sneak a peek at your medical chart.

Health care reform proposals that rely heavily on computerized heath data networks raise the ante on patient privacy. Health care reformers agree that the efficient collection, management, use, and storage of health data is critical to health care reform. Most foresee the eventual development of a comprehensive electronic health data network.

Most visions of a health data network feature an all-inclusive database of health and health-related information. Personal information about every citizen's prior illnesses, medications, allergies, and family health risks would be included, as would public health information, including patterns of illness and injury, expenditures of medical resources, experimental medical treatments, and public health risks. The system would be capable of storing and processing vast amounts of health information with unprecedented speed and efficiency.

The potential benefits of a health data network are impressive. Computerized medical records could lower costs, improve quality, and increase the accessibility of health care services. Some examples demonstrate the promise of this technology:

> **A**fter a skiing accident in Colorado, Steve undergoes surgery to stabilize fractures in his legs. There are complications when the surgeons are unable to control Steve's internal bleeding. Two seasons later, when Steve is run over by a snowblower, the surgeons anticipate the need to stock extra blood. They had learned of Steve's tendency to bleed from the health data network.

> **D**r. Egan, a gynecologist, gives each patient a sonogram at every visit, even at routine examinations. The insurance companies that cover Dr. Egan's patients learn about the doctor's testing practices by tapping into the health data network. In an effort to keep their costs down, the insurers notify Dr. Egan that they will not cover his patients for sonograms without proof that the tests are medically necessary.

> **M**ary needs bypass surgery. Five hospitals are located within a sixty-mile radius of her house, and she doesn't know which hospital to enter for the surgery. She refers to the hospital rating system of the health data network, and learns that The Pumper Pavilion has an A+ rating for cardiac surgery.

> **S**am went to see his doctor after back pain had been bothering him for a week. The doctor told Sam to relax (which only made Sam more agitated), and presented him with a $75 bill. Sam instantly filed his insurance claim through the data network. Previously Sam would have taken a month to get around to filing his insurance claim through the mail.

You get hit by a car and lose consciousness. Emergency medical personnel look in your wallet for identification, punch some numbers into a computer, and in a matter of seconds know that you had your tonsils removed when you were eight years old, you had gallbladder surgery last year, you drink a martini every day with lunch, are allergic to penicillin, and your father died of heart disease. This immediately accessible source of information enables them to give you better care at lower cost.

This is the good news. The bad news is that a database of health and related information may be available to individuals and organizations whom you would rather not have nosing around your medical files.

A potential employer, for example, might tap into the database to find out whether you are likely to take a lot of sick days. Or a professional adversary may enter the database looking for some incriminating information to use against you.

Organizations that conduct outcomes analysis already depend on large databases of patient information to do their job of identifying overutilized medical procedures and evaluating the effectiveness of different modes of patient care. These research organizations need massive amounts of data to identify trends of what works and does not work in health care. (See chapter 1 for more on outcomes analysis.)

The Federal General Accounting Office, recognizing the growing interest in outcomes analysis, recently issued a report that raised pressing concerns about the feasibility of protecting the confidentiality of patient-specific information once the information is pooled in these large databases.[75] Especially now that more and more outcomes data banks are maintaining patient-identifiable information, the threat to personal privacy is augmented.

Traditionally, much of the data collected by outcomes analysis organizations did not identify patients by name, but that is changing. Lawyers with an expertise in medical privacy expect that the time will soon come when patients who are harmed by unauthorized or improper disclosures of patient-identifiable information will have a right of action against outcomes researchers and the hospitals that provided the researchers with access to patient records.

Facsimile (fax) machines, which electronically transmit written information from one location to another, raise similar specters of lost privacy. In many ways, fax machines are a godsend to the health care industry. In the time it takes to make a telephone call, a doctor can now receive a wealth of written information about a patient's medical history and test results by fax.

While the obvious benefit of receiving information by fax is saved treatment time, the potential for a breakdown in confidentiality is equally clear. Electronic transmissions can be intercepted, mistakenly sent to unintended recipients, or picked up and read by anyone who happens to be standing at the fax machine when the transmission comes through.

Medical facilities, on the advice of their attorneys, are starting to take steps to prevent breaches in patient privacy when medical records are transmitted by fax. Hospitals may face legal liability if they fail to take such reasonable preventive measures as reconfirming the fax number before transmitting patient data, using cover sheets specifying that the information is confidential, and verifying that the faxed information has been received. Patients who are harmed by faxed information that falls into the wrong hands may also have legal recourse.

Can networks of stored data be secured so that access by unauthorized individuals is barred? There is reason to believe that the answer to this question is no, at least given the existing patchwork of federal and state laws that are in place to safeguard informational privacy.

The Institute of Medicine, a private group chartered by Congress, recently completed a study of the confidentiality of patient health data in the age of computers. The institute's report concluded that "The balance between the advantages of such databases and their potential for harm . . . is not yet clear." [76]

According to the report, current privacy laws fail to provide adequate regulation of computerized collections of medical records. There are several areas of vulnerability.

First, the existing laws do not impose the same stringent confidentiality requirements across the board. The required degree of confidentiality depends on several factors, including who controls the information, the type of information involved, and the relevant jurisdiction. These distinctions will be difficult to maintain once a range of health data, gathered across state lines, is compiled in an exhaustive database.

Second, current law barely addresses secondhand disclosures of confidential health information. Patients are left virtually unprotected if someone with legal access to confidential information makes an unauthorized disclosure of that information to a third party.

Third, many state statutes on informational privacy apply to manual patient records. Automated records may fall outside their purview.

Some privacy experts see that the solution to these problems lies in a sweeping federal statute that would replace the existing assortment of state laws. National uniformity is unlikely to be achieved without a comprehensive federal statute. A prior attempt by the National Conference of Commissioners on Uniform State Laws to establish a Uniform Health Care Information Act in 1985 failed. Only two states, Montana[77] and Washington,[78] ever enacted the act.

A uniform federal law would apply the same confidentiality requirements both inside and outside the health care setting. Health care providers who gather and record health data, as well as non-provider individuals and organizations who receive transmissions of health data, would be subject to the same confidentiality requirements. Proposed legislation would also afford the same degree of protection to all types of health information. The results of an HIV test would receive no greater protection than the results of a standard blood-type test would.

Finally, to ensure the confidentiality of the health data, proposed federal statutes on informational privacy would allow only specified parties access to the database. Individuals seeking information about themselves, parents seeking certain types of information about their minor children, legal guardians seeking information about their incompetent wards, approved researchers, physicians with their patient's consent, and physicians treating patients for life-threatening conditions could have access to the database. Non-authorized individuals could not access the confidential health information, with or without the patient's consent.

A new federal law, though certainly a boost to informational privacy, might not be enough. Additional safeguards may be required to protect the confidentiality of a database of medical information.

Some means of personal identification will probably be required. Just as a depositor cannot access his or her bank savings through an automated teller machine without a personal identification number, a patient, provider, or other interested party would not be able to access the health database without an appropriate identification number.

Social Security numbers might appear, on first blush, to be the logical choice for an identification number. Why give out new identification numbers when we each already have our own, unique, Social Security number?

Your Social Security number is already used to identify you in connection with such nonmedical matters as taxes, cable television, credit cards, education, employment, and driving licenses. With the widespread problem of forgery and theft of Social Security numbers, these and other such databases that are accessed through your Social Security number become virtually unprotected. If the Social Security number can also unlock the door to your medical records on the health data network, the threat to your privacy would be complete.

A new health identification number dedicated to the health database might provide enhanced security. Of course, a health identification number only goes so far in protecting the patient's privacy. Although outside "hackers" who do not have the identification number may be barred access to the protected data, authorized users could still wrongfully disclose the confidential information for money, revenge, or any other purpose.

PRIVACY AND MEDICAL TESTING

An individual's interest in maintaining the confidentiality of his or her medical records is perhaps most pressing when the record reveals a stigmatizing medical condition, such as substance abuse or infection with the HIV virus. How should the interests of society in tracking and treating these conditions be balanced with the individual's privacy interests?

Let's look at drug testing first. The most common types of drug testing utilize blood or urine samples. To collect a blood sample, the subject's skin is punctured. To collect an absolutely reliable urine sample, the subject urinates on demand under direct observation.

Given the havoc illegal drug use has wreaked on society, widespread drug testing is intuitively appealing. Why wouldn't we want to identify, attempt to rehabilitate, and monitor every drug user?

The problem is that drug testing intrudes on individual privacy. Both the collection of test samples and the potential for misuse of test results raise pressing privacy concerns.

In two landmark 1989 cases the U.S. Supreme Court upheld limited federal drug testing of railroad workers involved in accidents and Customs Service employees seeking promotions to sensitive jobs. In the course of considering the case, the justices expressed concern about the intrusiveness of drug tests into a fundamentally private domain. The tests passed constitutional muster only because the subjects of the tests worked in jobs related to public safety. Today, government employees who carry weapons or operate heavy machinery or vehicles are commonly subject to drug testing. Efforts to test public employees whose jobs are not related to public safety have been blocked by the lower courts.

In 1995, the High Court ruled for the first time on the constitutionality of random drug testing of student athletes. The American Civil Liberties Union had argued that urinalysis drug testing is so intrusive as to be unconstitutional without suspicion of drug use. The school district had argued that any invasion in student privacy was justified by the district's interest in curbing drug use. The Supreme Court held that public schools could require their athletes to submit to drug testing[79]

President Clinton recently announced a plan to seek drug tests for every suspect arrested on federal charges. Defense lawyers were quick to question the constitutionality of the plan.

Different rules apply to drug testing in the private sector. The Constitution only restricts government activities; it does not apply to private industry or individuals. In the private sector, drug testing is common regardless of the involvement of public safety. About 78 percent of large companies now test workers for drugs, which is nearly a fourfold increase since 1987. In many cases, prospective employees have no legal bases for objecting to a drug test.[80]

The absence of regulations protecting subjects of private drug testing programs is especially surprising given the potentially damaging uses to which these tests can be put. At the very least, disclosure of the results of a drug test can be embarrassing. Of far greater significance is the potential loss of employment, discrimination, and stigmatization.

Drug testing raises other privacy concerns as well. Tests of blood and urine samples can yield a wealth of information *other than* the presence or absence of a particular drug. For example, pregnancy, depression, diabetes, schizophrenia, heart trouble, and the use of contraceptives, can all be ascertained through blood or urine analysis. The nonconsensual discovery of these conditions raises troubling privacy concerns.

Adolescents understand the risks of seeking treatment for drug and alcohol abuse. A 1993 study found that privacy concerns are a significant deterrent to adolescents who might otherwise seek treatment for substance abuse. About 25 percent of the students surveyed said they would forgo health care if they thought their parents might find out the nature of the treatment.[81] An earlier study found that more adolescents—49 percent—would seek care for drug use if assured that the treatment would be confidential.[82]

The horrifying spread of AIDS raises new concerns about the privacy of test results. One question that has moved to the fore of public debate is whether there should be mandatory testing of all newborns for HIV infection. Those who favor a mandatory testing program point to the benefits of early intervention in the treatment of the AIDS virus. Those who oppose the testing point to the privacy interests of mothers. (Evidence that babies identified as HIV-positive would suffer discrimination from doctors is also sometimes cited in support of non-disclosure. Research has shown that newborns with the AIDS virus would have a 50 percent less chance of receiving cardiac surgery and would be far less likely to receive costly dialysis than their equally sick but non-infected counterparts.)

Forty-four states currently test babies for HIV for statistical purposes to track the spread of AIDS, but parents cannot learn the results of the tests. The question presently under debate is whether doctors should be required to notify parents of the results of HIV tests that are performed anonymously.

Although the benefits of receiving early treatment are obvious, the compelling privacy interests of mothers makes this question troubling to many people. Infected newborns cannot be identified without identifying the HIV status of the mother as well. Babies can only contract the virus from their mothers in the womb or at birth. Mandatory testing of newborns means, in effect, mandatory testing of mothers. At this time, only Federal prisoners can be tested for HIV without their consent. Some of the nation's most powerful lobbying groups—including AIDS activites, women's and gay groups, and civil libertarians—oppose mandatory testing and notification laws. With confidential testing, only the government knows the identity of the 7,000 babies born each year who are at high risk of developing AIDS.

The vigorous debate underway in New York State is illustrative. Since 1987 New York has required all babies to be anonymously tested for HIV. The names of the babies were not associated with the test results. In March 1995, a New York City advocacy group for children filed a lawsuit on behalf of HIV-infected children seeking to compel the state to disclose the test results. The group's motivation was clear. Infected infants stood a better chance of getting treatment if their mothers knew of their HIV status.

Attempts to resolve the lawsuit legislatively were unsuccessful. The Speaker of the New York Assembly blocked a vote on a mandatory testing and notification bill (succumbing, according to critics, to pressure from powerful lobbyists). Finally, in October 1995, state officials announced that the lawsuit had been settled. The results of the HIV tests would be made known to the familes of the infected babies.

Genetic testing, the latest addition to the medical testing arsenal, is raising new privacy concerns. These tests enable scientists to identify genetic predispositions to breast cancer, colon cancer, skin cancer, and thyroid cancer. Will insurers use these test results to deny or restrict coverage to people at high risk of developing cancer? Will employers deny jobs to genetically flawed applicants?

According to the federal Equal Employment Opportunity Commission's 1995 compliance manual, the use of genetic test results to deny employment could be considered discriminatory under the 1990 Americans with Disabilities Act. The government's top genetecist, the director of the Human Genome Project, has warned that federal legislative intervention is needed to protect from employment and insurance discrimination Americans who get tested for genes that indicate a susceptibility to certain diseases.

Seven states currently have genetic privacy laws. The U.S. Senate Cancer Coalition called hearings to debate the need for federal legislation after a 1995 study of families with inherited diseases found that 31 percent of the families had been denied insurance coverage, even if they were not ill.

ADOLESCENTS AND HEALTH CARE PRIVACY

Adolescents need privacy like flowers need water. An adolescent who has a private health concern, such as a drug problem, a sexually transmitted disease, an unwanted pregnancy, or depression may be primarily concerned about maintaining the confidentiality of his or her condition; receiving timely medical treatment may be of secondary concern. With adolescent morbidity and mortality on the rise, the medical profession has recognized the importance of providing adolescents with confidential health services.[83]

Traditionally, parental consent was required for the treatment of minors. Minors were presumed to lack the capability to make reasoned decisions regarding their care. Over time, the courts and state legislatures have chipped away at the parental consent requirement. Parental consent is still mandatory, but only under certain circumstances. (See chapter 2 for a complete discussion of informed consent.)

Sometimes a parent becomes involved in a child's medical treatment in connection with the payment of the doctor's bill. When the child is covered by the parent's private insurance policy, the parent receives a claims form in the mail itemizing the covered services. When the child is covered by public medical assistance (Medicaid), the youth must present the family's Medicaid card or documentation about the family's finances. Eighty-three percent of all adolescents are covered by private or public health insurance.[84]

Where the patient's privacy is within the doctor's control, the doctor must balance the parent's interest in the child's health and well-being with the patient's need for privacy. Neither the courts nor the legislatures have given physicians who treat adolescents much guidance.

Adolescents who are concerned about the confidentiality of their medical care should follow these recommendations:

➤ Ask the physician to describe the limits of the confidentiality of the doctor-patient relationship. The patient should be assured that the doctor will not disclose medical information without the patient's consent, except under the limited circumstances of a patient who threatens suicide or is unable to make reasoned health care decisions. The doctor and patient should agree on what constitutes a "reasoned health care decision." Any decision that is consistent with the patient's values and beliefs should be considered to be a reasoned decision, even if it does not conform to the decisions the doctor would make under similar circumstances.

➤ If the doctor and patient disagree about whether or not a parent should be informed, the doctor should either suggest ways for the adolescent to inform the parent on his/her own or offer to be present when the parent is informed. Doctors who are not comfortable treating a minor without the parent's consent are under no legal obligation to do so. The patient should find a new doctor.

➤ The patient and physician should discuss the payment arrangement in advance. If the doctor will be performing a confidential medical treatment or procedure, the patient should assume personal liability for the bill.

RESOURCES

If you have questions about the privacy of your medical records, the following advocacy organizations are good sources of advice and assistance:

Center for Medical Consumers
237 Thompson Street
New York, NY 10012
212-674-7105

Consumer Information Center
P.O. Box 100
Pueblo, CO 81002
Send $.50 to order the booklet Protecting Your Privacy *(stock #583A).* Your Right to Federal Records *(stock #368A) is free.*

Medical Information Bureau
P.O. Box 105
Essex Station
Boston, MA 02112
617-426-3660

Residents of Canada:
Medical Information Bureau
330 University Avenue
Toronto, CAN
MSG 1R7
416-597-0590

Request the free publication "MIB, Inc.: A Consumer's Guide," and "The Consumer's MIB Fact Sheet" and/or a copy of your file.

National Academy Press
2101 Constitution Avenue
Washington, DC 20418-0001
800-624-6242

Call for information about purchasing the Institute of Medicine's report entitled "Health Data in the Information Age" and the National Research Council's report "Computer Based Patients' Records."

The National Women's Health Network
514 10th Street, N.W., Suite 400
Washington, DC 20004
202-347-1140

Public Citizen Health Research Group
Dept. MR2
2000 P Street, NW, Suite 650
Washington, DC 20036
202-833-3000

Send $10 for booklet entitled "Medical Records: Getting Yours."

FOUR

Your Rights
as a Hospital Patient

Even if you never commit a crime, and never do time in jail, you may still wake up one morning at a time not of your choosing in a small room completely lacking in privacy, being offered rock-hard eggs, pasty white bread, and diluted orange juice. Then you'll remember. You were just admitted to the hospital.

Residents of medical facilities rival prisoners when it comes to loss of personal autonomy. Both populations are told what to do, and when to do it. Neither group has control over the food they eat, the clothes they wear, or the places they go. Hospital patients cannot lock the door to their room or freely schedule visits with friends and family. They are routinely spoken about in the third person, and are often referred to by their room number.

As an incoming hospital patient, the cards appear to be stacked against you. Something is amiss with your mind or body. You may be weakened by illness or debilitated by pain. You are probably feeling frightened and vulnerable.

Despite this less than rosy picture of hospital life, desperation and dependency need not rule the day if you find yourself facing a hospitalization. Hospital admissions do not have to turn confident and competent adults into fearful and dependent patients. The conversion from a position of strength to one of weakness is *not* inevitable.

Hospital patients have rights, and it is those rights that are the subject of this chapter. Read on to learn what you can do to protect your interests before, during, and after a hospitalization.

PATIENT RIGHTS AND ADVOCACY TIPS

Many patients receive a copy of the Patient's Bill of Rights when they enter the hospital. The Bill of Rights was drafted by the American Hospital Association in 1973 to protect patients in the hospital. Every accredited hospital must post the Bill of Rights in hospital corridors, and may provide a copy to incoming patients.

The rights of hospital patients as set forth in the Bill of Rights fall into three general categories—courteous treatment, privacy, and informed consent. The protections set forth in the Bill of Rights are summarized briefly below. Although some of the rights in the Patient's Bill of Rights are legally enforceable and can be the subject of a lawsuit, others are not legally binding on hospital administrators. A discussion of what you can do to protect your nonlegal Bill of Rights entitlements follows the summary below.

1. *The right to considerate and respectful care.* Courteous behavior is notoriously difficult to legislate. Your right to courteous treatment from hospital personnel, though not legally enforceable, can be the basis of a grievance if, for example, a doctor calls you "honey" or "sweetie" despite your objections, or neglects to pull the curtain around your bed during an examination after you have requested privacy.

2. *The right to complete information from your doctor about your diagnosis, treatment and prognosis in easy-to-understand language, and the right to know by name the physician responsible for coordinating your care.* This right is an aspect of the legally enforceable right of informed consent. Informed consent is covered in depth in chapter 2.

3. *The right to information about the specific nature of the proposed procedure and/or treatment, risks involved, medical alternatives, probable duration of incapacitation, and the name of the person responsible for the procedure and/or treatment.* This right, like the second right discussed directly above, is part of the legally enforceable informed consent doctrine.

4. *The right to refuse treatment, and to be informed of the medical consequences of your refusal.* The legally enforceable right to refuse treatment is part of our constitutional right of personal autonomy. This subject is covered in depth in chapter 6.

5. *The right to privacy concerning your medical care. Those not directly involved in your care must have your permission to be present during case discussion, examination, and treatment.* This right is premised in your legal protection against invasions of privacy. If you are a patient in a teaching hospital, this right may support your objection to being repeatedly scrutinized by unreasonably large and frequent gatherings of doctors and students around your bed. Rights of privacy are explored in chapter 3.

6. *The right to expect that all communications and records pertaining to your*

care will be treated as confidential. Once again, this reflects your legal right to sue a doctor or hospital that discloses information about your condition or treatment without your permission. Chapter 3 covers the right of privacy in its specific application to health care matters.

7. *The right to expect that the hospital will make reasonable efforts to respond to your request for services, and will not transfer you to another facility without first advising you of the need for the transfer and ensuring that the receiving facility will accept you for transfer.* The part of this right that deals with transfers is legally enforceable. A hospital breaks the law when it refuses to treat a patient that the hospital is equipped to treat if the patient's condition might worsen as a result of the hospital's refusal. Hospitals that lack the necessary staff or equipment to treat a patient are legally obligated to arrange for that patient's transfer to an appropriate facility. This subject is discussed in greater depth later in this chapter.

8. *The right to obtain information about relationships between the hospital and other medical and educational institutions, and relationships among individuals who are responsible for your care.* This right is intended to protect patients from conflicts of interest among their health care providers. You have a right to know, for example, if the hospital where you had surgery is owned by the same health care corporation that owns the rehabilitation facility to which you have been referred for postoperative care. This right also relates to the right of informed consent. (See chapter 2.)

9. *The right to information about proposed human experimentation affecting your care or treatment, and the right to refuse to participate in such research projects.* This legally enforceable right is part and parcel of the right of informed consent. Patients must consent to participate in medical research studies. They must be advised of the nature and risks of the research and their right to withdraw from the study at any time. (See chapter 2.)

10. *The right to expect reasonable continuity of care.* This right makes good medical sense. The quality of your care depends on knowing when you will be seeing a doctor, who that doctor will be, and what you should do between doctor visits. Your right to quality medical care is the subject of chapter 1.

11. *The right to examine and receive an explanation of your bill.* Few hospital patients have to fight for their right to *receive* a copy of their bill; getting someone to explain each charge to the patient's satisfaction is, however, another matter.

12. *The right to know what hospital rules and regulations apply to your conduct as a patient.* This commonsense right benefits hospitals and patients alike.

The protections embodied in the Patient's Bill of Rights are not self-enforcing. You must take affirmative steps to make sure your rights are protected.

WHEN YOU HAVE A COMPLAINT

If you believe one or more of your hospital rights is being violated, you may want to start by raising your grievances with the patient representative, advocate, or ombudsman.

Patient representatives or ombudsmen are on staff at many hospitals to serve as advocates for the hospitalized patients. Some hospitals assign an advocate to each newly admitted patient. The job of these advocates is to informally resolve patient grievances without resort to the courts.

There is a tremendous range of quality among patient advocates. Some advocates are truly dedicated to promoting the interests of hospitalized patients, while others are mere public relations tools for the hospital.

In all fairness, patient advocates employed by hospitals are in a difficult position. On the one hand, they are paid to help address patient complaints. On the other hand, the subject of most patient complaints is the hospital, the organization that also happens to pay the advocate's salary. The conflict is clear.

Ineffective patient advocates are unwilling to risk their jobs by criticizing or antagonizing their employers. They tend to mollify complaining patients with noncommittal assurances that everything will work out. Effective advocates, in contrast, listen to and investigate patients' complaints, make recommendations and/or referrals to the appropriate authorities, and report back to the patients.

Say, for instance, you want to take a look at your hospital medical chart. Perhaps you are motivated by simple curiosity, or you are considering a malpractice suit. You may be lucky, and the first nurse you ask willingly turns over your chart to you. Or perhaps your doctor quickly delivers the records for your perusal. But your request to view your hospital chart might be met with suspicion by the hospital staff. Your nurses and doctors could refuse to comply with your request. You may want to take up the matter with the patient advocate.

Some hospitals allow patients to view their records if certain procedures are followed. Your advocate should be able to help you negotiate the procedures. In hospitals that do not provide patients with their records unless required to do so by state law, advocates should be able to explain the nature of the restrictions to you.

Some states give patients access to hospital records but not doctors' records, or vice versa. Other states leave disclosure of medical records to the discretion of the provider, allowing providers to withhold records they believe would harm the patient. A number of jurisdictions restrict the patient's right of access to the records by permitting providers to disclose only those records that pertain to a lawsuit, allowing patients to examine, but not photocopy, their records, or requiring providers to make summaries of the medical records available to patients while keeping the records themselves off limits.

If you have sought access to your medical records through your patient advocate and your efforts have not been crowned with success, ask the hospital for a written denial of your request for disclosure. Whether or not you get the written denial, you may want to consider filing a formal complaint with the hospital's grievance committee.

If, after a reasonable period of time, you are not given access to your records, write a letter to the hospital administrator. Advise the administrator about the situation and your intentions to pursue legal action, if necessary, to obtain your record. Once again, wait a couple of months for a response. If your request is denied or no response is forthcoming, it may be time to seek legal representation.

Lawyers can sometimes gain access to medical records that are not available to patients themselves. Depending on the law in your state, the lawyer may have statutory access to the medical records. If this is not the case, the lawyer may still be able to obtain the records in connection with a lawsuit based on the hospital's failure to disclose the records or for medical malpractice. Of course, a lawsuit based on the provider's failure to disclose the records should be brought only if the withholding of the medical records violates some statutory provision, and a medical malpractice suit should be brought only if there is actual evidence of negligence.

Medical records maintained by Veterans Administration hospitals and other federal medical facilities fall under the purview of the Freedom of Information Act (FOIA) and the privacy act. As a general matter, these two pieces of federal legislation protect the patient's right to see his or her own medical records. The policies of some state hospitals also conform to the FOIA and privacy acts.

If you are receiving care in a public facility and would like to see your medical records, call the medical records department. An oral request to see your records may suffice, or you may be required to put your request in writing.

Once you make a request to see your records, you should receive a response within ten business days. If access is granted, you will be charged the cost of copying your records. Additional fees are prohibited. If you are denied access to your records, you may sue the relevant governmental agency in federal district court to compel disclosure.

Patient advocates are not qualified to handle every type of hospital-related complaint. Different types of complaints should be directed to different parties.

If you feel you are being overbilled, for example, you should contact your insurance company or the state attorney general's office. You should communicate concerns about unsanitary conditions, fire hazards, infection control, and other matters concerning hospital operations to the state department of hospital licensing (listed in appendix 9). Quality of care issues, such as the inadequate staffing of emergency facilities or the unavailability of a broad range of specialists, should be taken up with the hospital administrator or chairman of the hospital's board of directors.

Special considerations apply when you are dissatisfied with the quality of your medical or nursing care. These types of grievances should be taken up with the medical staff itself.

Every hospital has a hierarchy of doctors and nurses, as shown in the following chart. When seeking to resolve a quality-of-care complaint, move up the ladder of authority from level one to level five until you reach the person who is willing and able to address your concerns to your satisfaction.

Physician Hierarchy

Level One ....Interns or first-year postgraduate trainees
Level Two........................Residents or postgraduate trainees
Level Three.....................Chief residents
Level Four ....Chiefs of services (internal medicine, pediatrics, surgery, etc.)
Level Five ....Chief of medical staff or medical director

Nursing Hierarchy

Level One ....Staff nurse
Level Two........................Head nurse or charge nurse
Level Three.....................Nursing supervisor (for the unit or floor)
Level Four ....Director of nursing

There are a few general recommendations to keep in mind when filing any type of complaint. First, keep your cool. You will gain nothing by raising your voice, resorting to vulgarities, name-calling, or putting the hospital employee on the defensive. The greatest success comes to those who communicate their complaints calmly and rationally.

Second, pick your battles carefully. Complain every time your eggs are overcooked, or your medication comes a few minutes late, and you will be amazed at how quickly an entire staff of nurses can be struck deaf.

Third, assume the best of people. The hospital staff is probably doing everything possible to make your stay as pleasant and successful as possible. If you think about it, the staff has nothing to gain by making you unhappy. If something has gone wrong, don't be too quick to criticize or look for bad intentions.

Fourth, compliment before your complain. We all like to know that our efforts are appreciated. Before launching into a litany of what's wrong, take a moment to thank the worker for something that was done right.

A situation may arise and you may be unsure of whether or not to file a complaint. Is the wrongdoing really as bad as you think, or are your expectations unreasonable?

When it comes to gripes against the nursing staff, here are some guidelines to help you assess the legitimacy of your complaints:

➤ *Do the nurses come to your room frequently enough?* As a general matter, nurses should check in on patients that are not seriously ill once every few hours. Seriously ill patients should be seen as frequently as once every fifteen minutes. Ask your doctor how often the nurses should check in on you.

➤ *Do the nurses respond to your summons quickly enough?* You cannot expect the nurses to handle each and every request immediately, but you should receive a prompt response each time you ring the nurses' station. A nurse should either come to your room in person or verbally respond over the intercom.

➤ *Do the nurses spend enough time with you?* "Enough time" means as much time as necessary to inquire about changes in your condition, ask if you have any complaints or questions, and wait for your response.

➤ *Do you never see the same nurse twice?* Some continuity of nursing care is important. You should expect to see one or two of the same faces each nursing shift.

When your complaints about the nursing care are not being addressed by those within the nursing hierarchy, it is time to contact your primary physician. Your primary physician, whether a private doctor from the community or a staff doctor assigned to you, is ultimately responsible for your well-being. It is incumbent upon your physician to make every effort to improve the quality of your nursing care.

When your concerns relate to your doctor's fitness to practice medicine, the stakes go up considerably. Take immediate action if your doctor has liquor on his breath, shaking hands, memory or reasoning problems, or touches you in an inappropriate or sexual manner.

Start by filing a complaint with the patient representative or ombudsman and the hospital administrator. Clearly state what action you would like the authorities to take. Do you want another doctor to be assigned to your case? Would you like an investigation to be commenced? Are you ready to be transferred to a different facility? What must you receive in compensation in order to forgo a lawsuit? Perhaps you want the hospital and doctor to forgive your outstanding medical bills or reimburse you for your out-of-pocket expenses.

The quality of care you receive in the hospital is constantly being monitored by the hospital's quality assurance system. Every hospital must have an internal quality assurance review system to maintain high standards of care.

As part of quality assurance, hospital medical staff review selected cases on an ongoing basis to see that standards of care are being met. Doctors who are found to be rendering inferior care to their patients are monitored more closely.

If their performance does not improve, they may lose their admitting privileges. In extreme cases, they may be reported to the state medical licensing board and lose their license to practice medicine. (See chapter 1.)

You may also want to file a formal complaint with the appropriate governmental agency. Different agencies regulate different types of medical professionals. The Board of Medical Examiners regulates doctors, the Board of Nurse Examiners regulates nurses, and the Office of Occupational or Professional Licensing regulates technicians. (The medical and nursing licensure agencies in each state are listed in appendix 4.)

Any formal complaint about medical wrongdoing should include all the following information and materials:

➤ Your name, address, and telephone number

➤ The names and addresses of the hospital and the provider(s) that are the subject of your complaint

➤ The details of the alleged wrongdoing, including when and where it occurred

➤ The names and statements of any witnesses

➤ Copies of all relevant medical records and other documents

Upon receipt of your complaint, the regulatory agency should conduct an investigation to determine whether disciplinary action is warranted. The agency may recommend some informal resolution to the grievance, or it may appoint a hearing officer to collect and review the relevant evidence, take the testimony of witnesses, and issue a finding. If you are not satisfied with the hearing officer's decision, which may be a dismissal of your complaint, you are always free to pursue a malpractice case in court. (See chapter 1.)

As a general rule, hospitals share legal responsibility for acts of malpractice that are committed by doctors practicing medicine within the hospital's four walls. This rule of shared responsibility holds true even if the physician is an independent doctor from the community who is not on the hospital's payroll. When a doctor makes a mistake diagnosing or treating a hospital patient's condition, both the doctor and the medical facility where the doctor was practicing medicine may be sued.

In addition to pursuing these administrative and judicial remedies, you may think about filing a grievance with a medical trade organization such as the American Medical Association. The benefit of filing such a grievance is that you create a formal record of the facts underlying your complaint, which could prove beneficial if your complaint ever results in legal action. Grievances filed with medical trade organizations rarely, however, result in any disciplinary action being taken against the offending provider. Medical trade organizations exist to support and defend their members—doctors. They are not in business to criticize doctors or blemish the medical profession's reputation.

HOSPITAL EMERGENCY CARE

Patients who come to hospital emergency rooms for treatment are protected by a federal (and sometimes state) statute with a most unglamorous nickname: the anti-dumping act. Anti-dumping acts prohibit hospital emergency rooms from denying treatment to patients on the grounds that the patient cannot pay for the care or for any other reason.

Patient dumping, or the practice of refusing to treat patients with emergency conditions, is illegal under state anti-dumping laws and the federal Emergency Medical Treatment and Active Labor Act. (The federal legislation only applies to hospitals that receive Medicare funds, which includes most American hospitals.)

Before anti-dumping laws were passed, a pregnant woman experiencing labor pains and bleeding could be transferred from a private hospital emergency room to a public facility without first being examined or having her condition stabilized. Now, transferring a patient with an emergency medical condition from one facility to another without the patient's written informed consent, or without first providing an evaluation and stabilizing treatment, is illegal. Furthermore, transferring a stabilized patient to a facility that lacks the space and/or personnel to provide the patient with appropriate care, or failing to forward the patient's medical records to the receiving facility, is also illegal.

Every patient who comes to a hospital emergency room is entitled to a medical evaluation to determine whether he or she has an emergency medical condition or is in active labor. Any emergency medical condition must be stabilized before the patient can be transferred to another medical facility. Unstable patients and women in labor cannot be transferred unless they ask to be moved, or a doctor certifies that the medical benefits of being treated at a different facility outweigh the risks of the transfer because proper treatment is not available at the transferring hospital.

The mere existence of anti-dumping laws does not ensure that your rights as an uninsured or underinsured patient seeking care in a hospital emergency room will be protected. In fact, 24 percent of patients transferred to a public Chicago hospital from other hospitals were found to have been unstable when transferred. The mortality rate of the transferred patients was almost three times that of the patients who were not transferred.[85] A 1994 study of compliance with anti-dumping laws conducted by the Public Citizen Health Research Group also yielded disappointing results.[86]

You stand a good chance of prevailing in a suit against the hospital based on the anti-dumping laws if you can prove:

1. You had an emergency medical condition
2. Your condition was not stabilized
3. You were transferred or discharged from the hospital
4. You suffered harm as a direct result of the transfer or discharge

The stickiest element of proof is usually number two. Hospitals tend to argue that a patient with constant vital signs (blood pressure, pulse, and respiratory rate) is "stable." The courts, however, have applied a different definition of stable. They have looked at whether the patient's condition was likely to deteriorate as a result of the transfer. If the answer to this question is affirmative, the courts have paid less attention to the stability of the patient's vital signs.

Anti-dumping laws adopt a "strict" or absolute standard of liability. This means that the patient has to prove only the four elements listed above to win his or her case. The patient need not prove negligence, malpractice, or any failure to exercise a reasonable degree of care. The strict liability standard of proof is tremendously beneficial to the injured patient's claim.

Hospitals and doctors that violate the federal law against patient dumping are subject to serious penalties. They can be precluded from participating in the Medicare program, fined tens of thousands of dollars, or both. If a physician practicing in the hospital violates the law against dumping, both the doctor and the hospital will be equally liable for fines and expulsion from the Medicare program.

A patient who is dumped and is harmed as a result can also sue the hospital for compensation. The availability of a private cause of action under the federal anti-dumping act is important to health care consumers. A private cause of action allows the injured patient to sue the hospital for damages. Without a private cause of action, only public agencies could enforce the law. Unfortunately, the hospital industry's voluntary compliance with anti-dumping legislation has been spotty, and government enforcement of the laws has been lax.

If you should ever find yourself in an emergency room, make sure you get the care you need when you need it. Do not wait demurely in the corner of the waiting area while your child's fever rages, your leg bleeds, or your elderly parent grimaces in pain. Bring your needs to the attention of the nurses and receptionists who guard the "In" door to the emergency room. The goal is to draw attention to your situation while not being rude or antagonistic. You will gain nothing by losing your patience.

You could start by asking the nurse or receptionist about how long you can expect to wait to be seen. If the predicted waiting time is excessive, call your private physician. Your doctor may be able to meet you at the emergency room and expedite your care, or arrange for a meeting with the appropriate specialist.

If your private physician is of no help, call the next nearest hospital. Confirm that a physician is on-duty, and inquire about the average waiting time. A shorter waiting time in another hospital's waiting room may justify the time you will spend in the car en route to the other facility.

If your private physician is of no help *and* there are no other local emergency facilities, your best bet is to sit tight and maintain your composure. Ask to speak with the head nurse. Explain to the nurse why it is absolutely necessary for you or your companion to be seen as soon as possible. Listen to the nurse's response. Is the explanation for the delay reasonable?

To expect the head nurse to promptly usher you into the emergency room treatment area is to set yourself up for disappointment. The purpose of presenting yourself face-to-face with the nurse is to make your presence known. Check back with the nurse every fifteen minutes or so. Let him or her know you are STILL waiting.

Don't waste your time confronting the desk clerk. Although you may succeed in driving up your blood pressure a few points, that's probably all you will accomplish. The desk clerk's authority is limited.

When your wait is finally over and you are summoned into the emergency room, your problems are over. Or are they? If your spouse, significant other, parent, or child has the medical emergency, what are your rights? Can you insist on accompanying your friend or family member into the emergency room treatment area?

Few emergency rooms extend a welcome mat for visitors. With limited exceptions, emergency room personnel can refuse to give a patient's companion access to the treatment area itself. Extra bodies can get in the way of emergency room personnel, who must move quickly from patient to patient.

You can, however, insist on accompanying the patient into the treatment area if the patient is a small child,[87] mentally disabled child, patient suffering from dementia, deaf or mute patient, or patient who is otherwise unable to communicate (possibly because of a language or educational barrier). In these limited cases your presence may be required to speak with the medical personnel on the patient's behalf, and to provide the close supervision that might not otherwise be available.

If you are truly convinced that your presence is needed in the emergency room and the doors remain closed to you, ask to speak with the director of the emergency room. If you require assistance during normal business hours, you can contact the hospital administrator. Your own private physician may also be of some help in defusing the situation.

If all else fails, and only then, you may want to consider forcing your way in. This extreme measure should only be used as a last resort, because it may work against you. You do not want the emergency room staff to retaliate, even in a subconscious way, by providing inferior medical care or attention to the patient you care about.

OUTPATIENT (AMBULATORY) CARE

Many medical procedures that once required hospitalization can now be performed on an outpatient basis at ambulatory care centers. At an ambulatory care center, you park your car, enter the building, undergo the procedure, leave the building, get back in your car, and go home, all in the same day.

Thanks to advances in medical technology, the availability of same-day surgeries has skyrocketed in recent years. Some procedures that can now be performed in one day on an outpatient basis include cataract extraction, varicose vein removal, hernia repair, tonsillectomy, tubal ligation, breast biopsy, dilation and curettage (D & C), and some types of plastic surgery. Ambulatory care centers have begun to spot the landscape in unprecedented numbers.

Your doctor should be able to provide you with information about the availability of outpatient care. He or she should be able to tell you what outpatient services are offered, and why those services are adequate or inadequate to meet your needs.

If your doctor says a hospital admission is necessary, consider getting a second opinion from an independent consultant. The decision to enter a hospital is important enough to warrant spending some additional time and money getting another doctor's opinion. For all you know, your doctor may be recommending a hospital admission for all the wrong reasons. Perhaps he is being pressured by the local hospital to admit more patients, or is under personal financial pressure to boost his income, or is taking extraordinary and unnecessary precautionary measures out of fear of being sued for malpractice.

Even if you must enter the hospital for surgery, you may be able to shave a day or two off your hospital stay by having at least some of your presurgical testing done on an outpatient basis. Most patients scheduled for surgery undergo a battery of tests one to three days before the scheduled date of the operation. The purpose of the testing is to provide the doctors with a set of baseline data about organ and glandular functioning, sugar and cholesterol levels, and cardiac activity.

Insurance companies have, on occasion, refused to cover days of inpatient care devoted to tests that could have been performed far more cheaply on an outpatient basis. In these frugal times, insurance companies are under increasing pressure to take cost-cutting measures to ensure their financial survival. If you do have your presurgical testing done in the hospital, make sure those days of your hospital stay will be covered by your hospitalization insurance coverage.

Although outpatient care can save you time, money, and the assorted indignities of hospital life, it must be approached with caution. All ambulatory care centers are not created equal. Before you enter an outpatient facility for treatment, make a preliminary on-site visit. How does everything look? Is the facility clean and odor-free? Are the rooms private?

Also, feel free to ask questions. Some suggested lines of inquiry follow.

1. Is the facility accredited? Accredited facilities have voluntarily submitted to a review of their compliance with national health and safety standards. Although accreditation is not essential, it does indicate that the facility

has met certain criteria. The Accreditation Association for Ambulatory Health Care (AAAHC) and the Joint Commission on Accreditation of Healthcare Organizations (JCAHO) accredit outpatient care centers. If you would like information about accredited centers in your area, you can reach the Accreditation Association for Ambulatory Health Care by writing to 9933 Lawler Avenue, Skokie, Illinois 60077-3708; or calling 708-676-9610, or the JCAHO at One Renaissance Blvd., Oakbrook Terrace, Illinois 60181, telephone number 708-916-5600.

2. Is the facility licensed or certified by the appropriate state agency? Have any complaints been filed against the facility with the state agency? To get answers to these questions, contact the state department of health or the department of hospital facility licensing. These state agencies are listed in appendices 1 and 9.

3. Are the doctors who staff the center board certified? Physicians who hold themselves out as specialists in particular areas of medical practice should be board certified. Ask in particular whether the doctor who will be administering the anesthesia or sedation, if any, is trained and certified. (See pages 7-8 for information on verifying board certification.)

4. What happens if you do not recover enough to return home the same day as the surgery? Many centers have overnight accommodations or are affiliated with a local hospital. The staff of the ambulatory care center should be willing to call an ambulance for you, and make all other necessary arrangements to facilitate your transition to inpatient care. You should not be left on your own.

5. What happens if a medical emergency arises during surgery? The center should be staffed with nurses, technicians, and physicians who are trained in emergency services. Procedures should also be in place to speed your transfer to a nearby medical center that is equipped to deal with medical emergencies. Ideally, the center should be affiliated with a local hospital.

6. What happens if a medical emergency arises after the surgery is completed and you leave for home? Is there a twenty-four-hour number you can call that is staffed with trained professionals? Contingency plans should be in place.

Insurance carriers generally favor outpatient care over inpatient care. The reason is obvious: money. Inpatient care costs insurers a fortune. From the cost of the patient's room and board down to the last aspirin and Band-Aid, hospital bills build and build.

Never assume, however, that you are covered for ambulatory care. Make sure your carrier recognizes the outpatient care center that you intend to enter as one that is appropriate for performing the medical procedure you require. You do not want any unpleasant surprises when you file your claim for coverage down the road.

SELECTING A HOSPITAL

At the risk of sounding melodramatic, an admission to an inappropriate hospital can mean the difference between life and death. As the following examples demonstrate, some hospitals are better suited than others to treat certain types of patients and conditions:

➤ You are unable to stop coughing. If you go to a hospital that is staffed and equipped to perform advanced medical diagnostic tests and the latest nonsurgical medical procedures, you may be able to avoid costly and perhaps unnecessary surgery.

➤ Your eighteen-month-old daughter is sick with a viral infection and has a high fever. The hospital ten minutes from your home may not be equipped with child-size tubes to use for the intravenous feedings. A children's hospital, on the other hand, would certainly have them.

➤ You suffer from anorexia and bulimia. You are more likely to encounter professionals who are familiar with the medical and psychological aspects of your medical condition if you enter a hospital that specializes in the treatment of eating disorders.

Contrary to popular belief, you are not at the complete mercy of your doctor when it comes to selecting a hospital to enter for treatment. Although your doctor will refer you to the hospitals that have given him or her admitting privileges, you are free to enter a different facility. In deciding whether to accept or reject your doctor's recommendation of a hospital, consider your doctor's answers to the following questions:

➤ What does the selected hospital have that the rejected hospitals lack?

➤ How does the doctor know that the selected hospital is the "best" hospital for treating your particular medical condition?

➤ What does the doctor know about the relative recovery rates of different hospitals in the area?

➤ How many of the procedures you will be undergoing are performed in the selected hospital each year, and how does this number compare to other hospitals in the area?

➤ What are the sources of the doctor's answers to your questions?

If you think a hospital is a hospital is a hospital . . . think again. Hospitals fall into several distinct categories. There are specialty hospitals, general hospitals, teaching hospitals, and non-teaching hospitals. When and why would you want to select which type of facility?

Specialty hospitals admit only one type of patient or patients with only one type of medical condition. There are specialty hospitals that only admit children, patients with orthopedic problems, elderly patients, or patients with cancer. Most specialty hospitals are located in urban areas. Residents of many rural communities may never know a specialty hospital.

General hospitals, in marked contrast to specialty hospitals, are prepared to treat a wide range of patients and ailments. They have the staff and medical equipment to handle a larger variety of medical conditions. The staff of general hospitals are less focused in their experience and training.

If you accept the adage that practice makes perfect, you can understand why a specialty hospital is the place to go if you require highly specialized treatment of a complex or rare medical condition. A major study reported in the *New England Journal of Medicine,* for example, showed that the chance of dying from angioplasty is one-third higher at hospitals that perform only one or two of these procedures a week.[88] The explanation is obvious. The doctors, nurses, technicians, medical assistants, and other personnel that staff specialty hospitals develop an expertise in the limited medical services they provide day after day after day.

Highly trained physicians and scientists in the forefront of their field are drawn to specialty hospitals, where they are given the opportunity to practice with cutting-edge medical procedures and technology. Patients benefit from the expertise and experience of these specialists.

The obvious advantages of a specialty hospital are the qualifications of the staff and the caliber of the facility's resources. If you are being treated by a doctor who has privileges at a specialty hospital that treats your particular medical condition, consider yourself fortunate. Not only are you under the care of a highly qualified physician who has acquired prominence in his or her field, you are virtually assured of receiving first-rate care when you enter the specialty hospital.

While specialty hospitals offer hope to patients with complex medical problems or rare medical conditions, they are not for everyone. If you do not need the sophistication of a specialty hospital, you may find that patient quality of life is sacrificed to the facility's technical expertise. The staff of specialty hospitals are often criticized for neglecting and depersonalizing their patients. They tend to treat patients less like people and more like vehicles transporting interesting symptoms and diseases.

Many specialty hospitals also fall short when it comes to emergency services. A patient who is admitted to a hospital that specializes in the treatment of ear, nose, and throat conditions, for example, may go into cardiac arrest during reconstructive surgery. If the facility is not equipped to deal with cardiac conditions, the patient would have to be transferred to another medical facility after her condition was stabilized.

Both specialty and general hospitals can be teaching hospitals. Teaching hospitals have medical training programs for medical school students and graduates who are studying such specialized areas of practice as obstetrics, internal medicine, or surgery. Hospitals with teaching programs, or teaching hospitals, are different from non-teaching hospitals in several important respects.

In a teaching hospital, patients receive most of their care from the house staff. The house staff includes the doctors who are teaching the specialized clinical training programs, as well as the residents and interns who are participating in the postgraduate clinics. If a teaching hospital is affiliated with a medical school, patients also receive treatment from medical students.

The primary attraction of a teaching hospital is quality care. Teaching hospitals offer their patients the benefits of the latest medical know-how and newest medical technology. The staff of teaching hospitals are educating the next generation of doctors, so they must keep abreast of the latest medical developments. Hospitals that have residency programs undergo periodic review by outside organizations that monitor the quality of postgraduate medical training. Patients in teaching hospitals that are connected with a medical school benefit from the oversight of faculty members who supervise patient care.

The staff of teaching hospitals often include specialists such as internists, obstetricians, pediatricians, and surgeons, and super-specialists, such as liver specialists, infectious disease specialists, cancer specialists, diabetologists, cardiac surgeons, and vascular surgeons. Most teaching hospitals have the personnel to treat virtually any kind of medical or surgical disease of any degree of complexity.

Unfortunately for patients in teaching hospitals, new doctors cannot learn everything they need to know from medical textbooks and journals. They need hands-on experience. If you are a patient in a teaching hospital, you will soon learn that new doctors will get the practical experience they need by putting their hands on you.

If you love to be the center of attention, you may actually thrive in a teaching hospital. You will probably receive more attention than you ever imagined possible.

Interns and residents will pop into your hospital room with alarming frequency to question, poke, prod, and inspect you. Clusters of white-coated doctors will assemble around your bed to scrutinize and confer. You will be the subject of impromptu mini medical conferences.

The attention of large numbers of students, residents, and interns comes at a price. Patients at teaching hospitals often report feeling like guinea pigs or museum displays. For many patients, the process is humiliating and degrading.

There is not much you can do as a patient in a teaching hospital to enhance your privacy. The scrutiny you receive is the price of receiving care at a top-notch medical facility. If your medical condition does not require the sophistication of a teaching hospital, you may want to opt for the more personal touch of a non-teaching facility.

What if you live in a town that has no specialty or teaching hospitals? Your only choice is the small 250-bed local hospital or the 600-bed hospital in the nearest city. How do you know which hospital to enter if you require inpatient care?

In many rural areas, a small hospital is the only hospital. Patients who require only routine medical care, or emergency care before being transferred to a larger facility, can usually receive the care they need in a small hospital.

Most small hospitals are perfectly well equipped to perform such routine surgeries as hysterectomies, appendectomies, gallbladder operations, hernia repairs, cataract operations, and to treat such well-understood medical conditions as pneumonia, diabetes, hepatitis, and kidney infections. Certainly such common medical conditions as sprains, fractures, and minor infections can be treated adequately at almost any small hospital.

If you do not have a complex medical condition that requires the resources of a larger medical facility, you may well be better off seeking treatment in your small neighborhood hospital. Smaller hospitals are generally more personal. You are more likely to be referred to as "Mr. So-and-So," rather than "the appendectomy in Room 305." Other benefits include proximity to your loved ones and your personal physician's oversight.

Quality varies among small hospitals. If you plan to enter a smaller hospital, look for one that is owned by a public agency, large corporation, or for-profit hospital chain. These small facilities have the financial backing of a well-capitalized owner. Newer hospitals are generally better than the older facilities. Learn all you can about the hospital's reputation. Local doctors can often offer insights into the quality of medical facilities in the community.

Small hospitals are, however, frequently limited in the services they can provide to their patients. In many cases they lack the resources that are available to their larger counterparts. This disparity makes it difficult for the smaller facilities to attract high-quality medical professionals and purchase state-of-the-art medical equipment. Studies of vascular and cardiac operations, as well as pancreatic cancer surgery, have all found higher survival rates among patients treated at large, high-volume hospitals.

Traveling miles away from home to enter a sophisticated medical center for the treatment of a simple medical condition is like retaining Clarence Darrow to represent you in connection with a parking ticket. It's overkill. However, just as you would not want a first-year law school graduate defending you against murder charges, you probably do not want to go to a small hospital for brain surgery, an organ transplant, neonatal intervention, or treatment of extensive burn injuries.

Here are some additional tips for finding the hospital that is best equipped to give you the care you require:

➤ If possible, go to a children's hospital for the treatment of a child's health problems. The staff of a children's hospital are trained to address the unique needs of children, both medical and nonmedical. Radiologists on staff in a children's hospital, for example, have the necessary experience to locate a tiny fracture in a child's skull X-ray that might go undetected by a radiologist who works with the general population.

➤ If rehabilitation services will be required, make sure the hospital has a fully equipped physical therapy department that is staffed by trained therapists and overseen by a physician therapist. Do not undergo hip replacement surgery or an amputation in one facility if you know you will have to be transferred to another facility to obtain the necessary postoperative care.

➤ Specialty hospitals like Sloan Kettering in New York (cancer), Texas Heart Institute in Houston (cardiac), and other hospitals that specialize in neurosurgery, eye surgery, pediatric surgery, and liver diseases can be located with the assistance of the reference librarian at your local public library.

➤ One way to get the name of a facility that employs a doctor who has a special expertise treating your particular ailment is to read medical journals. Find out who has written articles pertaining to your medical problem, and research the author's hospital affiliations. (Medical research by the layperson is discussed in chapter 1.) Your state department of health is also a good source of information about hospital treatment specialties. (State departments of health are listed in appendix 1.)

➤ If you will be entering the hospital for surgery, find out how frequently the procedure you are slated to undergo is performed. Don't make the mistake of going under the knife of surgeons who perform bypass surgery once a month when another hospital a few miles away does weekly bypass operations. The American Heart Association guidelines suggest that hospitals should not offer angioplasty unless they perform at least 200 such procedures each year.[89]

➤ Pick a hospital that is accredited. Ninety-eight percent of all hospitals are accredited. Accredited hospitals have undergone a voluntary review by a non-profit organization called the Joint Commission for the Accreditation of Hospitals (JCAH). The JCAH is jointly sponsored by the American Medical Association, the American College of Surgeons, the American Hospital Association, and other national medical groups. Most accredited hospitals display the accreditation certificate in the lobby, admissions office, or some other public place. Accreditation is different from licensing. Accreditation is voluntary, but every hospital must be licensed. State agencies only license hospitals that comply with a variety of health, safety, and zoning regulations. (See appendix 9 for a list of state licensure agencies.)

➤ Pick a hospital that is clean, convenient, and well staffed. Advance notice of your hospitalization will enable you to call the volunteer or community relations department of the hospital to schedule a tour. Take note of any unpleasant odors. Is the waiting room neat and safe? What about the lobby? If your prospective visitors don't drive, make sure the facility is located within walking distance of public transportation. Strike up a conversation with some of the patients. What can they tell you about the quality (or lack thereof) of the food? The disposition of the hospital staff? The accommodations? What are your opinions of the staff? Are they generally pleasant, available, and willing to answer your questions?

➤ Pick a hospital that has a pharmacy, preferably one on each floor. A pharmacy on each patient floor offers the benefits of quicker service, greater involvement of the pharmacists in patient care, and the availability of pharmacists to answer patients' questions. Prescriptions should be transmitted to the pharmacy by computer or facsimile (fax). Pharmacists who rely on telephone conversations with nurses can fill a prescription for disaster if the nurse mispeaks or the pharmacist mishears a word.

➤ Pick a hospital that has special care units. The two most common special care units are intensive care and cardiac care units. Better facilities have well-equipped and well-staffed special care units to deal with especially complex medical conditions.

➤ Pick a hospital with a good nosocomial record. Nosocomial infections are infections that are acquired during hospitalization. They are caused by microorganisms that thrive in the hospital environment. Some possible sources of information about a hospital's nosocomial record include your referring physician, the local department of health (see appendix 1), and the hospital administration itself. A hospital with an active infection control committee is likely to be on top of the situation. Also, a hospital that has someone on staff who is a member of the Association for Practitioners in Infection Control (APIC) probably monitors nosocomial infections. (You can contact the APIC by calling or writing 1016 16th Street, NW, 6th Floor, Washington, D.C. 20036; telephone number 202-296-2742.) At the very least, the hospital you select should have at least one nurse-epidemiologist on staff for surveillance purposes.

➤ Pick a hospital that is reputed to have a caring and competent nursing staff. Do not underestimate the importance of hospital nurses. These health care workers do far more than fluff your pillows. They monitor changes in your physical and emotional condition, treat your illness or injury, carry out your medication regimen, offer support and encouragement, and address your quality of life concerns (such as overcooked food, chilly room temperatures, and noisy hallways). Studies show that recovery times drop as the quality of nursing care rises.

The attitude of a hospital's nursing staff generally reflects how nurses are treated by the hospital administration and staff doctors. Hospitals that treat their nurses with respect, encourage them to participate in patient care, and compensate them fairly often offer superior medical care.

Local nursing associations and nursing employment agencies can be good sources of information about the relative strengths and weaknesses of hospital nursing staffs. You can also ask the hospitals themselves for information about their nurses. Find the hospital with the most highly trained nurses, lowest percentage of part-time and temporary nurses, best nurse-to-patient ratio, and slowest turnover rate and you have probably found the hospital with the best nursing staff around.

➤ To get feedback from other patients who have been treated at the facility, contact your state health department and the facility itself. State health departments maintain records of patient complaints. (See appendix 1.) Also, many hospitals have on file questionnaires completed by former patients, which should be made available to you upon request.

If you become convinced that you would receive the best care at a hospital at which your physician does not have admitting privileges, you can decide to enter that hospital. There are, however, some advantages to entering the hospital by way of your personal physician's referral.

While you are in the hospital, you depend on your personal physician for just about everything. Not only do you need your doctor to provide you with the best possible medical care, but you also need your doctor to serve as your advocate.

Your private doctor can help resolve complaints you may have with the house staff. Say you are upset because the internists and residents are treating you like a pincushion. Your doctor may be able to persuade the staff to make more efficient use of each blood sample they draw from you. Your doctor may also be able to convince the staff doctors to be more forthcoming with pain-relieving medications. Sometimes hospital staff withhold painkillers out of fear of legal liability for adverse side effects and possible addiction.[90]

Independent physicians from the community are often more willing to go to bat for their patients against hospital staff and administrators than are staff doctors who are employed by the hospital and have their patients assigned to them. Not only do the community-based physicians have a preexisting relationship with, and presumably some loyalty to, their patients, but they are also not as beholden to the hospital as the staff doctors are.

Patients who want to enter a hospital that has not given their personal physician admitting privileges must present themselves for admission. If they are accepted, the hospital will assign a physician to them. The assigned physician will be a hospital employee or a private doctor with admitting privileges at the facility.

PAYING FOR HOSPITAL CARE

Much of the hospital admissions process is devoted to money. How do you intend to pay for your care?

If private insurance or Medicare will be covering your stay, you will be asked to sign a release giving the hospital permission to supply information about your treatment to the insurer. If you do not have public or private insurance, you may be asked to pay for your care in advance or be referred to a special office that will be able to help you apply for financial assistance.

Many private hospitals do not welcome requests for financial assistance. These facilities are profit-making ventures that are in business to make money. When the patient does not have private insurance, the hospital may require payment in advance.

Public hospitals, in contrast, do not require advance private payment. Social workers in these facilities will assist uninsured patients with applications for publicly funded medical assistance, charity care grants, payouts, bank loans, and/or alternative methods of payment.

Hospitalized patients who do not have adequate public insurance (Medicare) or private insurance typically look to Medicaid (Medi-Cal in California) for medical assistance. Medicaid is a joint federal-state public benefit program that is funded with tax dollars. Only applicants who demonstrate financial need qualify for Medicaid. Because of its low levels of reimbursement and the extensive paperwork involved in participating in the Medicaid program, some hospitals do not accept Medicaid coverage.

Despite the hospital's interest in getting paid, a law prohibits medical facilities from delaying tests and treatment to inquire about an incoming patient's method of payment or insurance status. (See preceding discussion of patient dumping.)

Whoever is paying your hospital bill will want to know that the bill is correct. Just as no one would want to pay for a cup of coffee the waiter forgot to bring to the table, so no one wants to pay for a CAT scan that was never scheduled. Unfortunately, reviewing a hospital bill for accuracy is no small feat. Line after line of coded entry must be deciphered, and every syringe, aspirin, and bandage must be recalled.

Even those gifted with a remarkable memory will have difficulty validating with complete accuracy all of the charges on their hospital bill. How do you know, for example, whether that vial of blood the technician drew on the first day of your hospital stay was the subject of ten tests or twenty tests; you only know you are being charged for twenty tests. You also probably have no way of knowing whether you were lying on a disposable mattress cover, much less what the cover cost. At best, you will be able to verify the big-ticket items: room charges, the use of operating rooms and special care units, X rays, CT scans, MRIs, and prescription drugs.

Hopefully your hospital stay will be covered in whole or in large part by insurance. Insurance coverage takes some of the pressure off when it comes to validating every item on your hospital bill. Of course, insurance companies should not be paying erroneous hospital charges either; insurers are, however, in a better position than yourself to absorb the cost of an extra urinalysis or barium enema.

Many insured hospital patients are surprised to learn that several thousands of dollars of their hospital bill are not covered by their insurance. If you are in the hospital billing office when you learn that you owe the hospital $8,000, don't worry. The hospital is well equipped to treat shock.

Insurance policies vary in their coverage of hospital care. Some pay a dollar amount for each day of hospitalization, others pay a percentage of the daily cost of care, and still others provide 100 percent coverage. Some pay up to a million dollar maximum, while others terminate after $5,000 of coverage. Some policies have a $500 deductible, some have a $5,000 deductible, some have no deductible at all.

If you have a dispute with your insurance company over the extent of your coverage, contact your insurance agent or broker. You should be able to get a copy of your policy and an explanation of your coverage. If you believe your insurer is guilty of some type of wrongdoing, write or call your state insurance department (listed in appendix 3).

The time to get your insurance coverage questions answered is **before** you require hospitalization. You should know the extent of your coverage and the consequences of every exclusion and limitation. Remember, a $5,000 limit on hospital coverage sounds generous enough until you realize that one day in intensive care can cost over $500. The $5,000 of coverage will be a drop in the bucket if you develop a serious illness that requires a multi-week hospitalization, surgery, and/or intensive care. Will you be able to afford to pay the uncovered portion of your hospital bill out of your savings?

You may want to look into purchasing "major medical" insurance if you do not already have it. This type of health insurance covers a single catastrophic loss from an accident or injury. Major medical policies can be purchased to supplement a standard health insurance policy.

Say your standard health insurance policy covers you for $5,000 of hospital care. Although this coverage may be adequate (barely) for your run-of-the-mill accident or illness, it will be grossly inadequate in the event of a serious medical condition. You might want to purchase a major medical policy to supplement your $5,000 of coverage. In the event of a serious illness or injury, the major medical policy would cover you for up to $500,000 or $1 million of related expenses.

Major medical insurance is usually a good idea if the maximum coverage available under your standard health insurance policy is less than $100,000. Standard policies that cap their benefits at $500,000 or a million dollars have major medical insurance protection built right in.

The cost of a major medical policy is relatively inexpensive. The reduced cost reflects the small likelihood that you will sustain a major injury or be diagnosed with a chronic or life-threatening illness. When you purchase major medical coverage, you buy the security of knowing that one catastrophic medical crisis will not wipe out a lifetime of savings.

Major medical coverage can be beneficial to Medicare beneficiaries as well. Medicare is the federal health insurance program for older and disabled Americans. Many Medicare beneficiaries supplement their Medicare coverage with a private Medi-Gap policy. Medi-Gap insurance, as its name implies, fills in the gaps in the Medicare coverage. For example, Medi-Gap insurance can be purchased to cover the Medicare deductibles and co-payments. A major medical policy can be purchased in addition to Medi-Gap insurance to cover expenses related to a prolonged illness.

CONSENT FORMS

Patients entering the hospital are occasionally asked to sign a blanket consent form. By signing such a form, they agree in advance to undergo a wide range of medical procedures during their hospital stay. (Informed consent is covered in depth in chapter 2.)

If you are asked to sign a blanket consent form, take comfort from the knowledge that these forms have not withstood judicial challenge. However, you should still resist inscribing your John Hancock on the form until you have at least requested permission to modify the form. If permission is granted, make a notation right on the form that by signing you are not giving up any rights that are otherwise available to you.

If you are denied permission to modify the form, consider asking to speak with a supervisor or hospital administrator. If these higher authorities also deny your request to modify the form, you should probably go ahead and sign the form as is. If push ever came to shove, the form would be unlikely to withstand judicial scrutiny. Medical providers are required by law to obtain the patient's signature on a specific consent form before commencing treatment—whether or not a blanket consent form is already on file.

Any specific consent forms that you may be asked to sign during your hospitalization should accurately state all of the conditions under which you are consenting to the procedure. Do not be afraid to change the form before you sign it.

You may, for example, want to note that your consent is conditional on one particular doctor, surgeon, or anesthesiologist performing the procedure. Or you may want to explicitly withhold consent to any surgical procedure that is performed by a resident or intern. (Even if you are hospitalized in a teaching hospital, you have the right to refuse to be treated by medical students, interns, or residents.) You may also want to withhold consent to the disposal of tissues or parts that may be removed from your body in the course of the medical procedure. Items removed from your body can provide critical evidence in the event of malpractice. (See appendix 6 for a specific sample consent form.)

HOSPITAL DISCHARGES

In the traditional hospital discharge, your doctor will let you know when you are well enough to return home. He or she will notify the hospital at least twenty-four hours in advance of your impending departure, and the hospital will process your discharge. When you receive the news that you will be going home, you will probably want to shake your doctor's hand, express your profuse gratitude, and start packing. Wait a minute. Take some time to discuss a few important matters with your doctor before bidding your final adieus.

You need guidance about your post-hospital needs. What activities can you resume, and when? What foods can you eat? What should you do if the pain, bleeding, or temperature returns? When can you expect to feel totally back to normal? Which medications should you take, and when? When should you schedule a follow-up examination with the doctor?

Federal law requires those facilities that accept Medicare reimbursement to employ discharge planners. They help patients leaving the hospital make a smooth and safe transition to their home or residential facility. Discharge planning is also mandated by some state hospital licensure requirements, the internal discharge planning guidelines of some hospitals, and the guidelines of the American Hospital Association. If you are not afforded the services of a discharge planner in connection with your departure from the hospital, you can rely on any of these sources of authority to compel the hospital to provide you with this valuable service.

Discharge planners are especially helpful to patients who require rehabilitation therapy or ongoing monitoring after their hospital stay. The planners should provide these patients with a list of local agencies or organizations, or put them in contact with an appropriate home care agency. Patients who are being discharged to a nursing home should receive the assistance of the discharge planners in locating and gaining admission to a suitable facility.

Hospital patients are protected against inappropriate discharges. A proposed discharge of a patient hospitalized for hip replacement surgery to a nursing home that does not offer specialized rehabilitative services is a typical example of an improper and illegal discharge.

When you leave the hospital against medical advice, you discharge yourself. The hospital has no right to hold you against your will, and will not attempt to do so. The hospital and medical staff must only advise you of the risks associated with a premature departure, and then you are free to leave.

Patients who leave the hospital against medical advice are commonly asked to sign an unauthorized departure form. Any patient of sound mind who refuses to sign the form cannot be involuntarily held by the hospital. A hospital that refuses to let a patient leave can be charged with false imprisonment, even if the patient has not paid an outstanding hospital bill.

When you leave the hospital against medical advice and sign the unauthorized departure form, you acknowledge that you are leaving the hospital despite your doctor's warnings. You also relinquish any right to sue your doctor or hospital for malpractice if your condition worsens.

Some lawyers advise their patients against signing the unauthorized departure form. Although it is true that the hospital must let you leave even if you refuse to sign the form, your insurance company might not accept your refusal with equal forbearance. You may risk losing your insurance coverage.

A better way to proceed is to sign the form, but first ask if you can make some minor modifications to the form. If allowed, write down an explanation of why you are leaving against medical advice. Do you believe you would receive superior care in a different facility? Must you attend to a family emergency? Do you have a serious outstanding complaint against hospital personnel? Also, note that you are signing under duress and do not waive your right to sue for any damages that arise after your self-discharge as a result of negligent acts committed during your hospitalization.

If you are not permitted to mark up the unauthorized departure form, and fear a loss of insurance coverage, sign the form. The courts have looked with great skepticism upon any form that purports to waive the right to sue for negligence. You should be able to bring a malpractice suit, if the facts support your claim, despite having signed the form.

RESOURCES

Center for Medical Consumers
237 Thompson Street
New York, NY 10012-1090
212-674-7105

The Center for Medical Consumers is an advocacy group for patients and their families. A subscription to the center's newsletter, Health Facts, *costs $21 (one year) or $34 (two years).*

Consumer Information Center
P.O. Box 100
Pueblo, CO 81002

For information about using the Freedom of Information Act and the Federal Privacy Act to obtain records from the federal government, you can order Your Right to Federal Records *for $.50. Send a check or money order payable to "Superintendent of Documents."*

Freedom of Information Clearinghouse
Public Citizen's Health Research Group
2000 P Street, NW,
Suite 700
Washington, D.C. 20036
202-833-3000

The Freedom of Information Clearinghouse offers assistance to individuals seeking access to federal documents or records. If you are having difficulty obtaining records under the Freedom of Information Act or the Federal Privacy Act, you can contact the clearinghouse to see if you qualify for assistance.

Patients' Rights Office
State Department of Mental Health

The patients' rights offices of state departments of mental health are good sources of information about the rights of hospitalized mental health patients. The Los Angeles County Patients' Rights Office has translated into more than twenty languages the rights of mental health patients hospitalized in California. You can call 213-738-4888 for a translation. (Some state departments of mental health are within the state department of health. Departments of health are listed in appendix 1.)

FIVE

Your Rights as a
Nursing Home Resident

The numbers are impressive.

U.S. Census Bureau reports indicate that the number of people over age sixty-five is ten times what it was in 1900. By the year 2030, the over-sixty-five population is expected to double again.

According to predictions made by the Federal Agency for Health Policy and Research, half of all women and one-third of all men turning age sixty-five in 1990 will spend some time in a nursing home.[91] For a couple turning age sixty-five, the odds that one of them will require long-term care in a nursing facility are about 70 percent.

People eighty-five and older are expected to comprise the fastest-growing segment of the elderly population in the next century. About 22 percent of people age eighty-five and older live in nursing homes.

The math is simple and the conclusion inescapable: Long-term institutional care is on the rise. We are far more likely than our grandparents or great-grandparents were to see the inside of a nursing home.

Fantastic advances in medical knowledge and technology have contributed to the rising rates of institutionalization among the elderly. The bacterial pneumonia that quickly ended the lives of our ancestors can now be easily controlled. We enjoy an extended life expectancy, but we are also at greatest risk of developing the types of long-term debilitating illnesses that may impair our ability to live independently.

We are also more likely to require institutionalization in a nursing facility as a consequence of the virtual extinction of the extended family. If we had reached our eighties in the '50s, we probably would have spent the latter years of our life residing in the same home as an adult child, grandchild, niece, or nephew. Now we are far more likely to live alone.

Geographic mobility, lean economic times, changes in the housing market, and a different social climate have also played a role in making the cohabitation of young and old family members increasingly rare. It is not unusual for a single family to be scattered from New York to California. When a family remains geographically close, it may only be able to afford a small apartment or single-family home. When the family can afford a spare bedroom, no one may be at home during the day, since women, the traditional caregivers, have entered the workforce en masse. Even potential caregivers who are at home during the day may not have grown up with the expectation of caring for an elderly family member and may be unwilling to make the necessary lifestyle changes.

This is not good news to the many of us who share a perception of nursing homes as a dreadful place to spend the final years of one's life. The news is not, however, all bad. Laws and regulations passed within the last decade on both the federal and state levels have improved the quality of care and quality of life of nursing home residents. The legal status of the nursing home resident has never been better.

This chapter is divided into two sections. The first section is devoted to the most far-reaching piece of federal legislation, the Nursing Home Reform Law. This ambitious law attempts to alter the very nature of institutional care in this country. The second section considers other legal remedies that may be available to aggrieved nursing home residents.

THE NURSING HOME REFORM LAW

In the 1980s, administrative efforts to deregulate the nursing home industry were afoot. Congress responded by commissioning a study on the state of nursing home care in America. The study, which was conducted by the National Academy of Science's Institute of Medicine (IOM), culminated in a report entitled *Improving the Quality of Care in Nursing Homes.*

The report cited gross inadequacies in the existing regulatory scheme.[92] IOM's critical report was the last straw. Two years earlier, the U.S. Circuit Court of Appeals had ruled that the prevailing system of inspecting nursing homes failed to safeguard residents against deficient care.[93]

In December 1987, Congress passed the Nursing Home Reform Law. The reform law was included in a much larger piece of federal legislation called the Omnibus Budget Reconciliation Act of 1987 (OBRA '87). The reform law clearly attempts to remedy the problems with the nursing home industry that had been previously identified in the IOM report.

The reform law, which touches upon virtually every aspect of nursing home care, applies only to nursing facilities that are certified to participate in the Medicare and/or Medicaid programs (so-called participating or certified facilities). More than 80 percent of American nursing homes are Medicare and/or Medicaid program participants. Nonparticipating facilities are only required to comply with state licensure laws and regulations.

The federal Nursing Home Reform Law exists in addition to an extensive array of state laws and regulations. The states, under the federal reform law, were required to pass their own enactments to implement the federal reform law on a local level.

State rules implementing the federal reform law can be *more* restrictive than the minimum standards set out in the reform law, but they cannot be *less* restrictive. For example, if the reform law requires facilities to provide residents with a minimum of thirty-days' notice of discharge, state law could require sixty-days' notice but not a mere ten-days' notice.

Every facility that is licensed to operate within a state must meet the applicable state-imposed standards. Where the state standards strengthen the federal standards, the licensed facilities must meet the state standards. Where the state standards track the federal standards, licensed facilities must meet the federal standards. As already mentioned, state standards can never be less restrictive than federal standards.

The standards governing nursing home care changed on October 1, 1990, when the reform act went into effect. After that date, the rights of nursing home residents to receive services that maximized their well-being and enhanced their quality of life became matters of federal law.

To ensure that the nursing home industry rose to the lofty standards set by the new law, the legislators included an uncompromising enforcement scheme. Public surveyors became charged with the responsibility of conducting frequent and detailed on-site investigations and reporting noncompliant facilities to the appropriate regulatory agency. Survey results are available to the public through the facility or the state's certification and/or licensure agency.

Gone are the days when a facility's compliance with various building, fire, and safety codes was the paramount concern of nursing home inspectors. Modern-day nursing home inspectors now look for compliance with the quality of life and quality of care requirements of the reform law. They get most of the information they need from the residents themselves, not from snooping around the building and grounds.

Consider, for example, the way today's surveyors approach food in the nursing home. The cleanliness of the grill and the heat of the dishwasher water are no longer the inspectors' sole concerns. Now the surveyors are making sure that the legal rights of residents to influence what, when, and how they eat are realized.

The surveyors are supposed to ask the residents: Is your food flavorful? Appetizing? Well-balanced? Served at the proper temperature? Is it cut, chopped, or ground sufficiently? Are second portions available on request? What about a hot alternative to the main dish? Are Kosher meals available? How are requests to change dining companions handled? Are you given an opportunity to participate in decisions about menus, dining room decor, and serving times? Are the menus posted in advance? How many hours pass between the evening and morning meals? Is there a bedtime snack?

Where a resident is not capable of answering the surveyor's questions, the surveyor must draw his or her own conclusions about the quality, quantity, and adequacy of the food and food service.

This attention to food service and selection is appropriate, given the important role food plays in the lives of nursing home residents. Not only is good food essential to quality of life, but also food-related issues can directly affect the resident's physical and emotional well-being. Residents are less likely to eat food that does not look tasty or is not presented nicely. Residents who do not eat cannot thrive.

A nursing home that receives an unsatisfactory rating from a surveyor regarding food or any of the other areas of regulation under the reform law is subject to a variety of punitive measures. State licensing agencies can select among a menu of possible remedies to address violations of nursing home law. These remedies range in severity from the proverbial slap on the wrist to the loss of an operating license.

Before passage of the reform law, the government had few means at its disposal to punish noncompliant nursing homes. Although the federal government could cancel the facility's eligibility for Medicare and Medicaid reimbursement, this punishment served no one's interests. Noncompliant facilities lost their certification, and residents lost their homes. The government had to find alternative accommodations for the displaced residents, which was not an easy task.

The reform law has given public agencies a variety of possible responses to nursing home violations, including monetary penalties, the appointment of a receiver (a qualified outsider to run the facility), and/or termination of the facility's Medicaid or Medicare participation. Although these penalties are not directly available to aggrieved nursing home residents, the residents can file complaints with public officials who are, in turn, empowered to discipline noncompliant nursing homes. (The availability of a private right of action under the reform law is discussed below at page 119. Tips for finding an attorney to bring a lawsuit under the reform law appear at page 122.)

The reform law is divided into several different parts, with each part devoted to a particular aspect of nursing home life. The sections that follow focus on the statutory provisions that govern quality of life and quality of care, the resident's bill of rights, physical and chemical restraints, rehabilitation, and transfer and discharge. The final section of the chapter explores other legal remedies that are available to nursing home residents.

QUALITY OF CARE AND QUALITY OF LIFE

The resident assessment system is the foundation of the reform law's quality of care protections.

Every resident is entitled to a comprehensive assessment of his or her functional capacity and medical condition when admitted to a nursing home and periodically thereafter. The goal of the assessment is to evaluate what daily activities the resident can and cannot perform, and the nature of the resident's physical and emotional ailments.

The assessment is the basis of the care plan. The care plan describes the resident's medical, nursing, and psychosocial needs, and explains how the facility intends to meet these needs. The resident and the resident's family or representative have a legal right to participate in the preparation of the care plan.

A new resident is admitted to a nursing facility. At the initial assessment, the staff learns that the resident loves to cook, prefers to bathe in the evenings, frequently needs to use the bathroom in the middle of the night, and has started to fall with increasing frequency. Her care plan provides for an activity program of supervised cooking, nighttime baths, installation of a bathroom night-light, and a strength-building exercise regimen.

Care plans should be specific, spelling out precise treatment goals and identifying who is responsible for carrying out those goals. For example, a care plan that requires a nurse's aide to take the resident for a daily fifteen-minute walk is preferable to a plan that merely recognizes the resident's need for regular strength-building exercises.

In the best of all possible worlds, the assessment and care plan work together to meet the legal requirement that every resident receive "services and activities to attain or maintain the highest practicable physical, mental, and psychosocial well-being..." In practice, of course, every nursing home does not provide the highest standard of care to every resident. To determine whether a facility is providing your loved one with the quality of care required by law, take note of the following four steps.

1. First, write down a brief description of the resident's status at the time of admission. Was the resident able to eat, dress, toilet, ambulate, and move from bed to chair without assistance? Was she willing and able to communicate and socialize with other residents and staff? How would you describe her mental state? What about her medical condition?

   This description will help you evaluate the appropriateness of the services provided to the resident soon after admission. Were they excessive (inserting a nasogastric tube in a patient capable of self-feeding), inadequate (failing to cue a resident with dementia to eat), or appropriate?

   A description of the resident at the time of admission also establishes a baseline to be used in the future to evaluate changes in the resident's status. Did the resident's functional abilities decline? Was there deterioration in her medical condition? Mental status? This information will be invaluable as you proceed on to step two.

2. The second step of the quality of care evaluation is to note changes in the resident's functional and medical status, and consider possible causes for the changes. Was development of the new medical problem inevitable, given unavoidable changes in the resident's physical condition? If not, what are the alternative explanations for the resident's decline? Did the facility respond to the resident's deterioration by conducting a new assessment and revising the plan of care? If not, make sure these steps are taken immediately.

3. Step three is to make sure the facility does everything possible to halt any further deterioration in the resident's condition. The new assessment should specify what must be done to maintain the resident at her current level of functioning and physical and mental well-being.

    Say you note that the resident has developed a problem with eating where no such problem existed before. The plan of care should be revised to require nursing home staff to encourage the resident to orally self-feed by offering tempting menu selections, a quiet dining environment, and cuing as needed. If the resident exhibits confusion, the assessment should include a reevaluation of the resident's medication regimen.

4. As a fourth step, make sure the facility is doing everything possible to raise the resident's functioning to its highest practicable level; a facility that just prevents a resident's further decline does not meet the legal standard.

    Take, for example, a resident who is losing muscle control. The facility should schedule sessions with an occupational therapist so the resident can learn new ways to hold a fork and toothbrush. A medical consultation with a specialist may also be beneficial to see if the patient would respond to changes in her medical treatment.

Contrary to what you might think, quality of life and nursing home institutionalization are not mutually exclusive. Nursing home residents who retain control over their lives can enjoy quality of life even after they enter a nursing home. Studies have shown that nursing home residents who are encouraged to assume responsibility for their well-being and who make choices about their care are more active and less depressed than residents who are not encouraged to participate in the decisions that affect their lives.[94]

The reform law requires every certified facility to "care for its residents in such a manner and in such an environment as will promote maintenance or enhancement of the quality of life of each resident." Toward this end, regulations implementing the quality of life section of the reform law refer specifically to self-determination and participation.

These regulations give nursing home residents the right to choose activities, schedules, and health care that are consistent with their interests, assessments, and plans of care. Residents also have the right to interact with individuals of their choosing, both within and outside the facility. They decide who they sit with at mealtime and who will enter their room for visits. They also have a legal right to make important decisions about their medical care.

The Health Care Financing Administration drafted interpretive guidelines that clarify how much control is enough control. Surveyors charged with the responsibility of enforcing the reform law are instructed to ask residents the following questions to assess facility compliance with the quality of life provisions of the reform law:

➤ Do you usually get up in the morning and go to bed at night at a time of your choosing?

➤ Is your sleep interrupted by anyone during the night? Why?

➤ Can you eat other than during scheduled mealtimes?

➤ Can you choose what you wear? How are you groomed?

➤ With whom do you eat? Is that your choice?

➤ If you want to visit with somebody, can you do it?

➤ If you need help getting somewhere, do you get it?

➤ If you want to leave the facility for short periods of time, can you do so?

➤ Can you spend your time in the facility pretty much the way you like?

The reform law, regulations, and interpretive guidelines are all drafted in recognition of the fact that a nursing home is far more than a medical institution. It is home to the residents who live in it. Residents of long-term care facilities have a legal right to exercise their individuality; they are not prisoners who have been institutionalized because of some wrongdoing.

In a scathing report published in the August 1995 *Consumer Reports*, researchers found the quality of care at thousands of nursing homes to be "poor or questionable at best"—despite the impressive standards of the reform law. Forty percent of all certified facilities were found to have repeatedly violated federal standards yet were permitted to continue operating.

NURSING HOME RESIDENT'S BILL OF RIGHTS

Nursing home residents have been protected under a federal bill of rights since the mid-1970s. The protections, however, have been embodied only in regulations issued by federal agencies, not in a statute enacted by Congress and signed into law by the president.

With enactment of the Nursing Home Reform Law, a federal *statutory* bill of rights came into existence. The federal statutory bill of rights joins many state nursing home bill of rights laws to protect residents of nursing facilities.

The bill of rights is not a wish list drawn up by nursing home advocates or an empty statement of good intentions from the nursing home industry. It is legally binding on all certified facilities. The owners and trustees of the homes must establish written policies that advance the legal protections set forth in the bill of rights.

Federal and state agencies are charged with the primary responsibility of seeing that nursing homes do not trample the rights of nursing home residents as those rights are defined in the bill of rights. Nursing home residents and their representatives can look to such public entities as federal and state regulatory agencies, the inspector general, the state attorney general, and the State Medicaid Fraud Control Unit to enforce the law on their behalf.

The reform law does not explicitly authorize residents to bring their own lawsuits against nursing facilities based on an alleged violation of rights. The extent to which the law *implicitly* authorizes private rights of action against nursing facilities is a matter of legal debate.

A full discussion of the legal arguments that support the finding of an implied private right of action is beyond the scope of this chapter. Suffice it to say that the legislative history of the law clearly manifests congressional intent to make private causes of action available to nursing home residents and their representatives,[95] and the courts have found an implied private right of action under the Nursing Home Reform Law.[96] Congress has also recognized that public oversight of nursing home standards affords residents inadequate protection.[97]

The federal statutory nursing home resident's bill of rights sets forth the rights and responsibilities of residents who live in certified nursing facilities. These facilities must make available to patients, their families, friends, sponsoring agencies, and representatives, and the general public a copy of the bill of rights.

The rights listed in the statutory bill of rights are fleshed out in other parts of the reform law and the Health Care Financing Administration's (HCFA's) regulations and interpretive guidelines. For example, the bill of rights guarantees residents reasonable advance notice of any transfer. Other statutory and administrative enactments specify the circumstances under which notice must be provided, mandatory contents of the notice, timing of the notice, and parties to whom notice must be furnished.

There are fourteen rights in the nursing home bill of rights. When the resident is incapable of understanding his or her own rights, the first four of the rights devolve to the resident's guardian, next of kin, representative payee, or sponsoring agency. Here, then, are the rights:

1. Every patient shall have the right to know and understand all of his rights and responsibilities as a patient, either before or at the time of admission and during the course of his stay.

2. Every patient shall have the right to be fully informed, either before or on the day of his admission and during the course of his stay, of all services offered by the facility, and of all charges not covered by Medicare or Medicaid, or the basic per diem rate.

3. Every patient shall have the right to be kept fully informed, by a physician of his choosing, of his medical condition unless medically contraindicated (as documented by a physician in his medical record), and be afforded the opportunity to participate in the planning of his medical treatment and to refuse to participate in experimental research.

4. Every patient shall be given reasonable advance notice of any transfer or discharge from the facility, and the right to be secure in the knowledge that such transfer or discharge will be made only for medical reasons, or for his welfare or that of other patients, or for nonpayment for his stay, except where prohibited by Medicare or Medicaid, and that all such actions be documented in his medical record.

5. Every patient shall be encouraged and assisted, throughout his period of stay, to exercise his rights as a patient and as a citizen. To this end patients are granted the right to voice grievances and recommend changes in policies and services to facility staff and/or outside representatives of his choice free from restraint, interference, coercion, discrimination, or reprisal.

6. Every patient shall have the right to manage his own personal finances, or to be given at least a quarterly accounting of financial transactions made on his behalf by the facility pursuant to his written delegation of this responsibility. Residents' funds must be deposited in interest-bearing accounts separate from the facility accounts.

7. Every patient shall have the right to be consistently free from mental and physical abuse, corporal punishment, seclusion, and free from chemical and, except in emergencies, physical restraints imposed for discipline or convenience, except as authorized in writing by a physician for a specified and limited period of time or when necessary to protect the patient from injury to himself or others.

8. Every patient shall have the right to be guaranteed confidentiality of all treatment and both medical and personal records and the assurance that these will not be released without his approval except as required by law or third party contract.

9. Every patient shall have the right to be treated with consideration, respect, and full recognition of his dignity and individuality, including privacy in treatment and in care for his personal needs.

10. Every patient shall have the right to be assured that he will never be required to perform services for the facility that are not included for therapeutic purpose in his plan of care.

11. Every patient shall have the right to associate and communicate privately with persons of his choice, and send and receive his personal mail unopened, unless medically contraindicated (as documented by his physician in his medical record).

12. Every patient shall have the right to meet with persons and groups of his choice and to participate in any commercial, religious, and community activities unless medically contraindicated (as documented by his physician in his medical record).

13. Every patient shall have the right to keep and use all of his personal clothing and belongings as space permits, unless to do so would infringe upon rights of other patients, and unless medically contraindicated (as documented by his physician in his medical record).

14. Every patient shall have the right, if married, to be assured privacy for visits by his or her spouse; if both are inpatients in the facility, they are permitted to share a room, unless medically contraindicated (as documented by the attending physician in the medical record).

Although each of the rights enumerated in the bill of rights is important, a few merit special attention.

First, let's look at the rights that relate to quality of life—perhaps the most difficult rights to safeguard. Take, for example, the right to be treated with consideration and respect in full recognition of one's dignity and individuality. There is an inherently subjective element to this right. Who's to say how much respect is enough?

Say you visit your loved one in a nursing home. To your dismay you find that her room smells musty, her hair is pulled back in a ponytail instead of being properly groomed in her accustomed style, and the nursing home staff calls her by her first name (which she would have hated). What avenues of recourse, if any, are available to you?

Start by informally approaching the nursing home staff. Share your concerns with them. If possible, convey a sense of confidence that the problems can be resolved easily and amicably. Take pains not to portray the problems as insurmountable, or put the staff on the defensive.

If the staff is not approachable, ask to speak with a supervisor (the "head nurse" or "charge nurse"), the director of nursing, and the nursing home administrator—in that order. Again, try to make your complaints known without accusing anyone of wrongdoing. Make it clear that you hope everyone can work together to promote the best interests of the resident.

If your efforts at informally resolving the problems are not fruitful, inquire about the facility's formal internal grievance procedures. Many nursing homes have resident councils and family councils to help maintain harmony inside the facility. When filing a grievance with the institution, use the standards set out in the bill of rights to help formulate your complaint. (See resources at end of chapter for sources of information about resident councils.)

You should also contact the state or local ombudsman. Every state office on aging is federally mandated to create an ombudsman program to "investigate and resolve complaints made by or on behalf of older individuals who are residents of long-term care facilities." Every state has at least one full-time ombudsman (see appendix 2). Many cities and counties also have a local ombudsman.[98] The ombudsman is the nursing home resident's advocate.

The ombudsman's job is to negotiate with nursing facilities in an attempt to informally settle grievances filed by residents and resident representatives. Ombudsmen have the legal authority to enter the premises of nursing facilities that are the subject of grievances, but they do not have legal authority to compel the facilities to take remedial action. The ombudsmen can only forward complaints to the relevant state agency with a recommendation of sanctions.

Another office to contact with a complaint against a nursing home is the state licensing and certification office. This office is usually a division of the state health department (see appendix 1).

State offices of licensure and certification inspect nursing homes to ensure that they meet all relevant federal and state standards. Facilities that are out of compliance with the laws and regulations may be found to be operating illegally. A facility will be more protective of residents' rights if it fears that its good name with the state licensing agency may be sullied.

If you are interested in taking legal action against a facility, contact the office of the state attorney general. You may also want to speak to an attorney on your own. To get a referral to a state or local legal services program that provides free legal assistance to older adults, you can call the Area Agency on Aging Eldercare Locator at 800-677-1116. Other sources of referrals to private attorneys who concentrate in nursing home law are the Nursing Home Litigation Group of the American Trial Lawyers Association (202-965-3500), the National Academy of Elder Law Attorneys (602-881-4005), and your local bar association.

In addition to a private right of action under the reform law, there may be other causes of action that are available as well. Where the resident has been physically or verbally assaulted by nursing home staff, a state elder abuse statute may be applicable. Elder abuse laws protect older adults from both physical and phychological mistreatment. A staff member who insists on addressing a resident by her first name over the repeated objections of the resident or resident's representative may be guilty of verbal abuse.

State consumer protection laws may also apply. A facility that holds itself out as a provider of quality care may be liable for fraudulent misrepresentation if there is proof that residents are actually subjected to unpleasant living conditions. Where the living conditions are intolerable, as opposed to merely unpleasant, an action for breach of implied warranties of habitability may also be available.

A second entitlement in the bill of rights that warrants special attention is the right to participate in one's own medical care. Residents and their legal representatives have the right to select an attending physician, even if the facility has staff physicians and even if medical services are included in the basic rate. This right also presents implementation challenges.

Many physicians make it a practice to stop treating a patient once the patient enters a nursing home. The physician's reluctance to treat the patient in a nursing home can have any number of origins. Some doctors want to avoid scheduling problems, others fear inconvenient nursing home policies, and still others are unwilling to accept the low Medicare and Medicaid reimbursement rates that may apply.

Some residents are willing to switch physicians once they enter a nursing home. They start receiving their care from a doctor affiliated with the nursing home, or a doctor recommended by their departing physician.

Residents who want to compel their physician to continue treating them after institutionalization can, however, get some help from the law. One general legal principle requires physicians to use, in the treatment of their patients, a reasonable or ordinary degree of skill and care. A physician who abandons an institutionalized patient by not returning the patient's telephone calls or not arranging to visit the patient in the facility may breach this duty.

A lack of the requisite diligence on the physician's part in attending to the patient's post-institutionalization needs constitutes negligence or malpractice. Where the negligence or malpractice causes an injury to the patient, the physician may face legal liability. Courts can levy monetary damages against physicians who wrongfully stop treating patients, when the patient worsens as a result of the physician's inappropriate withdrawal.

Physicians should continue treating their patients until one of the following events occurs: The doctor and the patient (or the patient's legal representative) end their relationship by mutual consent, the physician is dismissed by the patient (or the patient's representative), the physician's services are no longer needed, or the doctor gives the patient adequate and reasonable notice of his or her withdrawal. A physician who suddenly becomes unavailable to a patient following the patient's institutionalization may break his legal, and surely breaks his professional, obligations to the patient.

Where the doctor has provided advance notice of his or her withdrawal, the adequacy and reasonableness of the notice will depend on the prevailing circumstances. If the patient is in the midst of a medical crisis, the physician's notice of immediate withdrawal may not be reasonable. A notice of withdrawal that gives the patient one week to find another physician might be reasonable where the patient has the skill and opportunity to use a telephone, but unreasonable if the patient is confused and confined to bed.

Even where the doctor is willing to continue treating the resident in the nursing home, other problems may arise. The facility may not approve the physician for a staff appointment or give the physician guest privileges to treat residents on-site at the nursing facility, or the resident may be unwilling or unable to assume the additional expense of retaining the services of an outside physician if medical services are included as part of the basic rate. Even residents who go outside the facility for their medical care usually have to pay the same basic rate.

A third important right in the bill of rights empowers residents and their families to organize and join advocacy groups. This right gets its "teeth" from reform law provisions that give specified public officials from the Department of Health and Human Services, ombudsman programs, and state regulatory agencies immediate entry into certified nursing facilities. With the resident's consent, these public employees also have immediate access to the resident and the resident's medical records.

The availability of this type of public oversight helps residents and their representatives corroborate suspicions and substantiate complaints concerning the facility. Without the help of experienced public officials, residents and their families would have neither the time, experience, nor means to investigate and document institutional abuses and violations. Their right to form advocacy organizations would be an empty right.

The rights in the bill of rights that relate to money management offer the nursing home resident a double benefit. Not only do they protect the resident against pilfering, they also enhance the resident's sense of independence. Older adults who lose control over their finances often suffer from depression and feelings of helplessness and hopelessness.

Every nursing home resident on Medicaid receives a $50 monthly personal needs allowance. If the resident's only source of income is Supplemental Security Income (SSI), the personal needs allowance is paid by SSI. If the resident has other sources of income, such as Social Security or pension income, the resident is allowed to retain the allowance from these sources of income.

Residents use their personal needs allowance to purchase goods and services that are not included in the facility's basic daily rate. Typically the allowance is used to buy newspapers, stamps, candy, public transportation, and clothing. The personal needs allowance should not be spent on such essentials as soap and tissues, which should be provided by the facility at no extra charge.

The unspent portion of the resident's personal needs allowance accumulates month after month. The nursing home resident has the right to decide who will have access to, and control over, the personal needs account. The appointed money manager can be a friend, family member, or the nursing home. The resident is *not* required to keep the funds on deposit with the facility. Competent residents, of course, are free to open a bank account in their own name for purposes of holding the accumulated funds.

USE OF PHYSICAL AND CHEMICAL RESTRAINTS

Nursing home residents have been threatened with the use and misuse of physical and chemical restraints for decades.[99] They sound deplorable, but what exactly are physical and chemical restraints?

Physical restraints include any contraption that is attached on or near the resident for the purpose of restricting her freedom of movement or her ability to reach parts of her body. Examples of physical restraints include leg and arm straps, hand mitts, vests, wheelchair safety bars, and chairs with locking lap trays. An ordinary bed sheet can also be a physical restraint when it is wrapped around a seated resident's waist and secured behind the back of her chair.

Chemical restraints are psychoactive drugs, such as Haldol, Thorazine, Mellaril, and Valium, when these drugs are used to control behavior. "Unnecessary drugs" is another term for chemical restraints.

Although physical and chemical restraints are often discussed in the same breath, there are important distinctions between the two methods of control.

The use of physical restraints is readily apparent. These restraints are physically evident to the naked eye. Furthermore, their intended purpose is always to confine the resident. Leather straps that are used to bind a resident to her wheelchair, for example, never have a therapeutic objective.

The use of chemical restraints, on the other hand, cannot always be readily identified. Also, drugs that may have the effect of subduing a resident are not necessarily chemical restraints. They may be therapeutic. Psychoactive drugs are often appropriately prescribed to treat insomnia, depression, anxiety, and serious mental illness.

There is no way to identify a chemical restraint without knowing whether the patient (or representative) gave informed consent to the use of the drug, and whether the primary purpose of the drug is therapeutic. A patient who voluntarily takes a drug to control his hallucinations is not subject to a chemical restraint, even if the medication has the effect of sedating the patient.

Sometimes therapeutic drugs *become* chemical restraints. A drug that is initially administered to control a patient's medical symptoms becomes a chemical restraint when it starts to be used for the purpose of controlling the resident's behavior. Where the drug is administered for discipline or convenience, in excessive doses, for excessive periods of time, without adequate monitoring, or in a manner that results in a decline in the resident's functional status, it becomes a chemical restraint.

The pressures on nursing home employees to resort to restraints are undeniable. Restraints guarantee immediate behavioral control with minimal investments of time and energy on the part of the nursing home staff.

Many residents hit, swear, spit, wander, and/or scream out of fear, loneliness, or boredom. When the nursing home staff has neither the personal nor institutional resources to identify and remedy these anxiety-provoking emotions, they may look to restraints for help. Restraints bring difficult residents under immediate control.

Nursing home residents who are at greatest risk of being restrained are those who suffer from dementia. Dementia is an organic disorder that impairs the patient's memory, orientation, judgment, and thought processes. It affects up to

50 percent of nursing home residents. Studies have found that cognitive impairment is the greatest predictor of the use of restraints.

Nursing home residents with dementia frequently have communication difficulties. They cannot tell an aide that they are hungry, so they yell instead. They cannot express their desire to take a walk, so they flail their legs. They are most likely to be disruptive, both to staff and other residents. Restraints readily control these types of behavior.

Patients with dementia also often cannot understand the nature or purpose of proposed medical treatment, so they may be uncooperative and noncompliant. Restraints make it easier for nursing home staff to complete medical and personal care procedures.

Residents with dementia are also less capable of assessing the dangerousness of a situation. Staff are more likely to secure these residents in one place in an attempt to minimize the risk of injury from falls and wandering.

One of the primary benefits of nursing home reform has been the dramatic reduction in the use of physical restraints. According to the American Health Care Association, a trade group for nursing homes, fewer than 20 percent of nursing home residents are physicially restrained today, compared with the over 40 percent who were restrained in the mid-1980s.

Although the use of restraints is on the decline, some nursing homes still restrain their residents. The use of restraints is usually defended as necessary to protect the resident's safety, to protect the facility from legal liability, and/or to keep the facility's operating expenses within budget. The soundness of each of these proposed justifications for the use of restraints is examined below.

Restraints are sometimes needed, the nursing home industry has argued, to protect resident safety. This is a myth. There is no scientific evidence to support the claim that restraints protect nursing home residents from injury. In fact, there is evidence to the contrary.[100]

Residents who are restrained are *more* likely to sustain injuries than are their unrestrained counterparts. Restraints that are applied too tightly can cause bruises, blisters, and circulatory problems. Restraints that are too loose leave the resident at greater risk of falling and breaking a bone or sustaining a concussion.

When a restrained resident falls he is more likely to sustain an injury than when an unrestrained resident falls. A resident who slips through a physical restraint, for example, may become entangled in the restraint. In the worst-case scenario, he may choke to death in a desperate effort to extricate himself from the device.

Nursing home administrators also defend their use of restraints by citing a fear of litigation. They charge lawyers with laying in wait for an opportunity to sue nursing facilities for negligence. Once again, the perception that the use of restraints reduces the likelihood that a nursing facility will be involved in malpractice litigation does not withstand scrutiny.[101]

A review of the relevant case law shows that facilities that use restraints face a *greater* risk of being involved in malpractice litigation. What's more, facilities that restrain residents are also at greater risk of *losing* the malpractice cases they defend.[102]

A third argument in support of the use of restraints is premised on budgetary constraints. Nursing homes contend that they cannot afford to hire the additional staff needed to care for difficult residents. This argument is both illegal and unsound. Illegal, because the Nursing Home Reform Law and regulations require nursing facilities to employ sufficient staff to meet their residents' needs as a condition of certification. Unsound, because facilities that reduce or eliminate the use of restraints do not lose—in some cases they even save—money.

Nursing homes incur considerable expense when they use restraints. Most of the expense is attributable to the stringent regulations that require nursing homes to frequently monitor and attend to restrained residents.

At a minimum, nursing home staff must check in on each physically restrained resident at least once every thirty minutes. For ten minutes every two hours of restraint the staff must give the resident an opportunity to go to the bathroom, take a walk, and change position. The staff must also assist any restrained resident with a safety, comfort, or elimination need, and examine the resident for such restraint-related problems as skin and circulatory problems at every dressing and undressing session. Chemically restrained residents must likewise be monitored continually for the first thirty minutes and every fifteen minutes thereafter to detect and treat any adverse side effects. Nursing home employees must also maintain detailed careful records of restraint usage and monitoring schedules.

Committing so many staff hours to restrained residents can become very costly to a nursing home. The responsibilities associated with caring for restrained residents are mandatory and time-consuming.

Costs associated with the use of restraints continue to mount as restrained residents become less capable of self-care. Residents who are oversedated often lose the ability to dress or feed themselves. They require additional assistance. Similarly, residents who become weak after being tied to their bed can no longer walk to the bathroom by themselves. They must buzz an aide every time nature calls.

Restrained individuals are more likely to become incontinent. Incontinence alone costs the nursing home industry over $3 billion a year. Preventable pressure sores that result from being left in one position for too long add another $1.2 to $12 billion to the annual tab.[103]

The continued use of restraints is not justified by any of the rationales cited by the nursing home industry. Even if the rationales *were* sound, which they are not, the use of restraints should still be discouraged based on medical evidence of their potential for harm.

Physical restraints have been linked to cardiac stress, skin breakdown, muscular atrophy, upper respiratory problems, urinary tract conditions, constipation, incontinence, diminished appetite, dehydration, pneumonia, and injury from falls. Chemical restraints can cause a loss of muscle tone, infections, urinary incontinence, an inability to urinate, drowsiness, disorientation, and an enhanced risk of falls. With chronic use, chemical restraints can impair neurological functioning and result in twitching, slowed-down thinking and talking, confusion, imbalance, and repetitious behavior (such as licking lips).

An estimated 200 deaths a year are attributable to the use of restraints.[104] Restraint-related deaths are most often due to strangulation, contractures, and pressure sores.

The psychological impact of the use of restraints can be equally destructive. Restrained residents often suffer from social isolation, dependency, and a complete loss of self-esteem. Negative feelings of anger, fear, frustration, shame, and depression overwhelm many restrained residents. The residents often withdraw into themselves, stop eating, or develop sleep-related problems.

Of secondary concern is the effect the use of restraints can have on other residents in the facility, nursing home staff, and visitors. Residents of the facility who witness the use of restraints often become frightened. Staff become demoralized, and tend to treat the residents with less respect. Visitors who are shocked by the spectacle of a restrained resident may be discouraged from making return visits to the facility.

Despite the formidable risks associated with the use of restraints, it would be hasty to conclude that restraints should be prohibited under all circumstances. There are some limited circumstances under which the use of restraints may be justified.

A nurse needs to remove an intravenous line. If she does not remove the line and clean the site, an infection is likely to develop. The patient does not understand the nature of the procedure and resists the nurse's touch. Should the patient be temporarily restrained so that necessary medical treatment can be completed?

What about a nursing home resident who suffers from dementia and exhibits violent behavior? Other residents on the floor fear her outbursts. Should she be restrained to protect the other residents? Does the potential benefit to her floor-mates justify the risks of restraint?

Answers to these questions, and more, can be found in the reform law and its implementing regulations and interpretive guidelines.

The reform law implicitly discourages the use of restraints. The law's mandate to the nursing home industry to help each resident attain and maintain the highest practicable level of functioning and quality of life is inconsistent with the widespread use of restraints. Nursing homes do not help residents maximize their potential and avoid further decline by strapping them to their beds or doping them up with stupefying drugs.

The Nursing Home Reform Law also explicitly restricts the permissible use of restraints. Residents have the legal right "to be free from ... any physical or chemical restraints imposed for purposes of discipline or convenience and not required to treat the resident's medical symptoms." Restraints may be legally applied only under the limited circumstances set forth in the law.

The law allows restraints to be used to ensure the physical safety of the resident or other residents, and then only upon the written order of a physician. They may be used in an emergency situation for up to twelve hours without a physician's written order only where necessary to alleviate an immediate and serious danger to the resident or other individuals in the facility. Emergency orders authorizing the use of restraints must be confirmed in writing as soon as possible.

The use of restraints is illegal where less restrictive alternatives are available. Less restrictive alternatives to physical restraints include such supporting devices as pillows, pads, foam wedges, removable lap trays and rehabilitation therapy designed to prevent contractures and achieve proper body position, balance, and alignment. Therapeutic interventions that should precede the use of chemical restraints include environmental changes and attention to the resident's mental, physical, and psychosocial needs.[105]

Before any restraint is employed, the resident (or representative with legal authority to make health care decisions on the resident's behalf) must be told by nursing home personnel in a care planning conference about the intended use of the restraint. Care planning conferences are scheduled every three months or more frequently if the resident's health changes. At the conference, the nursing home staff, the resident, and the resident's family discuss all aspects of the resident's medical and nonmedical needs and care.

The nursing home staff must disclose to the resident or representative the risks associated with the use of restraints, including incontinence, decreased range of motion, decreased ability to walk, symptoms of withdrawal, depression, and reduced social contact. The resident (or representative) must then be asked to consent to the use of the restraint.

Representatives of nursing home residents have an important role to play in the care planning conference. They have a legal right to actively participate in the decision-making process that surrounds the use of restraints.

To evaluate the propriety of the proposed restraint, start by looking at the *likelihood* that harm will befall the unrestrained resident. Is the resident at high risk of falling if not restrained? Is she likely to develop a medical problem if left unrestrained? The lower the likelihood of harm, the less justification for the restraint.

Next, consider the *magnitude* of the potential harm the unrestrained resident faces. Is it minimal, like, for example, the risk associated with the disruption of an intravenous line, or is it life-threatening, as with the displacement of a ventilator's endotracheal tube?

If the magnitude of the risk is small, consider withholding consent. The known risks of using the restraints might outweigh the potential risks of *not* using the restraints. The nursing home staff may be inconvenienced by your decision, but that should not be your primary concern.

Also consider the anticipated duration of the restraint. Short-term restraints used for the purpose of completing medical treatment are more easily justified than is chronic restraint of patients who are difficult-to-manage.

The resident's likely reaction to the restraint is obviously a major concern. Some patients appear to be oblivious to restraints; others become extremely distressed or depressed. Of course, if the resident is unable to effectively communicate her emotions, you may not be able to use outward appearances as a reliable guide.

The resident's representative must also consider what steps the nursing home staff has taken to avoid the need for restraints. Have they designed an individualized restorative program to address the resident's underlying needs? Restorative programs can include exercise regimens to help a resident retain her strength, or social programs to lift a resident's spirits. Have they made changes to the resident's room to make the accommodations as safe and pleasant as possible? Is the furniture arranged so that the resident can easily get from the bed to the bathroom without tripping over an end table? Has the staff been educated about the resident's special needs? Have nonrestrictive supporting devices been attempted?

Restraints should not be used except when there are no less-restrictive alternatives available. If wandering is a problem, perhaps the nursing home could provide either diverting nighttime activities or a rocking chair, or install an individual door alarm or cloth barrier. For patients at high risk of falling, the home might be able to arrange for the bed to be closer to the floor, make bedside toilet facilities available, or locate the patient near the nursing station.

Homes that make liberal use of less restrictive alternatives to restraints can often be identified on an on-site visit. Look for building modifications that are designed to accommodate the special needs of residents who are most at risk of being restrained. Some facilities, for example have a "wandering loop." Wandering loops let restless residents amble around the interior of the facility without encountering any harm, locked units, or door alarms.

What happens if, despite all of these legal and procedural protections, a resident is wrongfully restrained? What avenues of legal recourse, if any, are available?

Residents who are wrongly restrained have their choice of possible causes of action under the law. They can sue the offending facility based on the implied private right of action under the federal reform law (see page 119), breach of contract, breach of implied warranties, and violation of state consumer protection laws.[106] Whatever cause or causes of action are selected, the nursing home is likely to mount a vigorous defense. One frequently employed legal defense strategy is to characterize a supportive device as an "enabler" rather than a restraint. Counsel for defendant nursing homes have been known to argue that the facility used a waist belt to "enable" the resident to sit upright in a chair; not to restrain the resident. Other facilities profess to be restraint-free because they only employ "reminder belts" or "safety belts"—not restraints.

Along the same vein, an attorney representing a nursing facility might argue that a device is not a restraint because it is secured by Velcro, not a knot or buckle. Although straps secured by Velcro may not be a restraint to the attorney, they may well be a restraint to a nursing home resident who lacks the mental acuity or physical strength to separate the adhered straps.

Any judge worth his or her salt should be able to see through these types of arguments. The relevant inquiry must always be the resident's freedom to move. Whatever benign term the attorney for the nursing facility may choose to substitute for the inflammatory "R" word, the rules and regulations that govern restraints should apply if the device is used to effectively control the resident.

What if a nursing home, at the time of admission, asks an incoming resident (or representative) to sign a document consenting in advance to the use of restraints? Is that legal? And what if the facility also asks the resident (or representative) to sign a document that releases the facility from liability if the resident is injured as a result of the use of restraints? Is that legal?

Probably not. The document that asks the resident to consent to the future use of restraints is likely unenforceable because it requires the resident to relinquish the important legal protections of the reform law. Although individuals are generally permitted to voluntarily waive their legal rights, they are not always permitted to waive legal protections that advance public policy. Legislative regulation of the use of restraints reflects the public's interest in protecting nursing home residents.

The document that releases the facility from future legal liability would probably also fail. Nursing homes are required by law to provide their residents with a high standard of care. Nursing home residents cannot defeat legislative intent by contractually consenting to some lesser standard of care.

What if a nursing home resident is threatened with an involuntary transfer or discharge from the facility if he or she refuses to consent to the use of restraints? Once again, the resident's legal position is strong. As discussed below, involuntary transfers and discharges are permitted only under limited circumstances. Refusal to be restrained is not one of the permissible grounds for transfer. Accordingly, the transfer of a resident who exercises her right to withhold consent to restraint would be illegal.

REHABILITATION SERVICES

The reform law manifests a clear legislative intent to transform the fundamental nature of long-term nursing facilities from custodial institutions to rehabilitation centers. Nursing homes must now make available to each resident specialized rehabilitation services that allow that resident to "attain or maintain the highest practicable physical, mental, and psychosocial well-being."

Nursing home advocates were thrilled to see this provision included in the final version of the legislation. They were all too familiar with the nursing home industry's lousy track record when it came to providing rehabilitative care.

Hospitals used to bear primary responsibility for providing patients with rehabilitative services. Nursing homes were neither expected nor equipped to be the frontline providers of rehabilitative care.

All this changed with implementation of Medicare's prospective payment system (PPS). Medicare hospital reimbursement stopped being available when a recovering patient could receive rehabilitation services outside the hospital setting. Hospitals became eager to discharge patients as quickly as possible, often to nursing homes for continuing treatment.

Before long, evidence started to mount that nursing homes were providing rehabilitative services inferior to the care that had been provided by hospitals. Before PPS, patients were receiving rehabilitation services in the hospital and being discharged directly home; after PPS, they were being admitted to nursing homes and remaining there for extended periods of time.[107]

The reform law was designed to improve the quality and availability of rehabilitation services in nursing facilities. Nursing homes must now provide residents with specialized rehabilitative services that "meet professional standards of quality." Physical, occupational, and speech therapy must be made available to residents whenever a "medical necessity" for the services exists.

In defining medical necessity, drafters of the reform law looked to a judicial interpretation of the Medicare statute. The interpretation arose in the context of a legal dispute over an institutionalized Medicare beneficiary's entitlement to covered therapy services where the beneficiary's condition was unlikely to improve with or without therapy. The court ruled that Medicare had to cover maintenance therapy services, even where the patient showed no potential for improvement.[108]

The reform law adopted this standard for determining a nursing home resident's entitlement to therapy services. Facilities must provide residents with therapy services that are needed to "attain *and maintain*" (italics added) the "highest practicable . . . well-being." Under the law, residents who need rehabilitative care to maintain their current level of functioning are as entitled to the care as are those residents who have a potential for medical improvement.

Consider the following two nursing home residents. Sal has degenerative arthritis. He already uses a walker and will never recover the ability to walk independently. He requires the services of a physical therapist to keep him out of a wheelchair for as long as possible. Bea is recovering from a hip fracture. She needs therapy so she can resume ballroom dancing. Both residents are equally entitled to therapy services in the nursing home: Sal to achieve his maintenance goal and Bea to achieve her rehabilitative goal.

When selecting a nursing home, you want to find a facility that takes its responsibility of providing liberal therapy services to heart. A federal study found that the percentage of residents enrolled in therapy programs ranged from about 0 to 50 percent among homes that offered specialized therapy services. Facilities that had the highest number of full-time registered nurses and that employed their own therapists (rather than contracting out rehabilitation services) were found to enroll significantly more patients in daily therapies and to discharge more patients home.[109]

TRANSFER, DISCHARGE, AND BED-HOLD POLICIES

The provisions of the reform law that apply to transfer and discharge are of critical importance to every nursing home resident. Studies have repeatedly shown that the trauma of a forced relocation to new living accommodations often causes extensive mental and physical setbacks in the older adult.[110] The legislators of the reform law took the risk of so-called "transfer trauma" seriously.

Transfers and discharges are also extremely trying for the family and friends of a nursing home resident. Placing a loved one in a nursing home once is tough enough; having to find alternative accommodations and resettle your loved one can border on the unbearable.

The reform law lists six circumstances under which involuntary transfers and discharges are allowed:

1. The resident's welfare cannot be safeguarded in the facility, and the transfer is motivated by concern for the resident's welfare.

2. The resident's health has improved so much that the facility's services are no longer required or appropriate.

3. The resident endangers the safety of other individuals in the facility, as certified by a physician.

4. The resident endangers the health of other individuals in the facility, as documented in the patient's clinical record and as certified by a physician.

5. The resident does not pay for an item or service not covered by Medicare or Medicaid that the resident requested, and the nonpayment continues after reasonable and appropriate demand for payment. (Transfer or discharge under this exception may not be permitted where the charge is being disputed, an appeal of a denial of benefits is pending, or if funds are not accessible. Funds may not be accessible where the resident is incapacitated and the court has not yet appointed a conservator or guardian.)

6. The facility stops operating.

Even if transfer or discharge is allowed under one of the six circumstances described above, the resident is entitled to at least thirty days' advance notice. The notice must identify the state long-term care ombudsman, explain the reason for the transfer/discharge, the scheduled date of release, the location to which the resident will be transferred/discharged, and information about appealing the facility's decision.

Depending on state law, exceptions to the thirty-day notice requirement may apply when the resident poses an immediate danger to the health or safety of others, requires urgent medical attention outside the facility, has resided in the facility for less than thirty days, or has experienced improved health. Under these limited circumstances, notice must be given as soon as practicable and an expedited discharge is allowed.

Family members and legal representatives known to the facility are also entitled to advance notice of the resident's impending release. They have the right to be informed about the facility's intentions, the reason for the proposed transfer or discharge, and precisely how and when the resident's departure from the facility will occur. The facility must work with the resident and the family to ensure the resident's safe and orderly release.

Despite these legal protections, facilities have been known to resort to illegal and deceitful practices to "unload" undesirable residents. Perhaps the most vulnerable class of undesirable nursing home patients are those who pay for their care with Medicaid, as opposed to private funds or private long-term care insurance. Nursing homes generally favor private-pay residents over Medicaid-covered residents because Medicaid pays the homes a lower basic rate than the private-pay rate. With the Medicaid residents, the homes get paid less for providing the exact same goods and services as they provide to the private residents.

Any attempt by a nursing facility to involuntarily release a resident based on the resident's method of payment is illegal. The law protects Medicaid-covered residents from this type of discrimination.

Some nursing facilities have attempted to circumvent the law by commencing transfer proceedings when a resident converts to Medicaid after his or her private funds are depleted. The home may fraudulently claim that the resident requires emergency hospital care, or poses a danger to himself or others, to bring the resident within one of the statutory exceptions to the prohibition against involuntary discharge or transfer. Residents and their representatives must be alert to these types of deceptive practices.

Nursing facilities also have an interest in discharging residents with behavioral problems, so-called heavy care patients. The involuntary discharge of this class of undesirable nursing home residents is also illegal.

Federal law permits nursing homes to discharge difficult residents only where there is proof that the facility cannot safeguard the welfare of the resident and others in the facility. Hard-to-care-for residents cannot be involuntarily discharged simply because they are difficult to supervise. The release of such residents violates the reform law, and may also run afoul of the federal Rehabilitation Act of 1973, the Americans with Disabilities Act, and the Civil Rights Act of 1964.

Even where the proposed transfer truly fits within one of the exceptions allowed in the reform law, residents (and their representatives) need not throw up their hands in defeat and accept the unwanted release as inevitable and unavoidable. Proposed transfers can be challenged in a court of law.

A judge who is presented with the right evidence may see fit to stop a proposed transfer dead in its tracks. One piece of particularly compelling evidence is a written statement from the resident's attending physician saying that transfer would not be medically safe, given the patient's physical and or mental condition. The court may also consider evidence that the discharge plan does not adequately address the patient's needs, or that no alternative care is actually available within a geographic area that would ensure the continuation of the patient's regular pattern of visitation. Finally, a judge may block a proposed transfer if presented with evidence that the facility could take alternative measures short of transfer to protect the safety of the patient and other residents in the facility.

Residents and representatives challenging a threatened or actual involuntary transfer or discharge should not overlook state law. Help may be available under the state consumer rights, contract laws, and/or common law duty of care, tortious abandonment, and intentional infliction of emotional distress.

A quick note about the opposite scenario: A nursing home resident wants to leave but is prevented from departing by the facility administrator.

A nursing home administrator cannot hold a resident who has not been adjudged mentally incompetent against her will, even if the resident's departure is against medical advice. The administrator is, however, responsible for warning the resident about the risks of leaving the facility. A resident who has been found to be mentally incompetent by a judge may be involuntarily institutionalized.

Not every release from a nursing facility is permanent. Sometimes residents temporarily leave a nursing facility to be hospitalized for treatment of an acute medical condition or to visit a family member.

These types of temporary nursing home departures are also regulated by the reform law. So-called bed-hold policies promote stability and predictability among nursing home residents.

Take, for example, a nursing home resident who is in poor physical health. She must be admitted to the hospital for treatment of her pulmonary condition at least once every couple of months. What would happen if, after every brief hospitalization, this patient lost her nursing home bed?

At best, she would be able to relocate to a comparable nursing facility. At worst, no bed would be available in a comparable facility and she would have to be temporarily maintained in inappropriate quarters. Under either scenario, the patient would likely suffer from the disruption to her routine and the unfamiliarity of her new surroundings. The risk would be a deterioration in her mental and physical functioning.

Bed-hold policies vary from state to state. In California, for example, facilities must offer seven days of bed-hold, while Illinois facilities must continue treating as a resident any patient who is hospitalized for up to ten days. In Florida, private-pay beds will be held for thirty days (as long as the nursing home continues to be paid), while Medicaid beds are held for up to fifteen days.

The federal reform law requires nursing facilities to provide residents with written notification of the rules governing temporary absences. Facilities are also legally required to accept Medicaid payment for holding a bed, and to give priority on readmission to Medicaid residents whose Medicaid-covered bed-hold has expired.

Nursing home residents who receive Medicaid are even guaranteed readmission if their temporary departure exceeds in duration the state's guaranteed bed-hold term. These residents must be readmitted to the facility following a temporary departure as soon as a bed in a semi-private room becomes available.

THE FUTURE OF THE NURSING HOME REFORM ACT

This book was in its final stages of production when both houses of the U.S. Congress drafted bills to repeal the tough provisions of the reform act. The Republican legislators indicated their intentions to shift responsibility for regulating the nursing home industry away from the federal government and onto the shoulders of state governments. The bills would have allowed the states to set and enforce their own standards for nursing home care, standards that could be much less stringent than those set by existing federal law. The proposals appear to have been scrapped, at least for now.

OTHER ASSORTED LEGAL REMEDIES

The first section of this chapter examined legal remedies that are available under the Federal Nursing Home Reform Law. This section considers other sources of law that also protect the rights of nursing home residents.

COMMON LAW DUTY OF CARE

As already discussed, nursing homes are bound by the statutory standard of care set by the reform law. There is an additional common law (judge-made) standard of care that nursing homes must meet at the risk of facing legal liability. Although the common law duty of care incorporates the standard of care mandated by the reform law, the two standards of care are not always identical.

The common law duty of care is defined by the degree of care that other facilities in the same geographic area exercise. A facility that complies with the statutory standard of care but falls short of the standard of care set by other nursing facilities in the area may be guilty of negligence.

Take, for example, a facility that physically restrains a resident. The resident becomes entangled in the restraint and is injured. Her family sues the facility for damages under the statutory and common law standards of care.

At trial, the defendant submits evidence that the restrained patient was checked every thirty minutes, as required by the reform law. However, the plaintiff presents evidence that the custom in local nursing homes is to look in on restrained patients every fifteen minutes. What is the facility's legal exposure?

Although the facility would not be liable for failing to meet the statutory standard of care, it may be liable for failing to meet the common law standard of care if the patient's injury resulted from the less frequent monitoring. The attorney for the nursing home could argue till she was blue in the face that her client complied with the relevant statutory and regulatory requirements, and the plaintiff might still win.

Now let's change the example a little. The facility, instead of looking in on the physically restrained resident every thirty minutes, only checked in once an hour. Now the facility is in violation of the statutory reform law and the common law duty of care. In some jurisdictions, a violation of the reform law is an *automatic* violation of the common law duty of care.[111]

Let's change the example one last time. The facility looked in on the restrained resident every fifteen minutes, consistent with local custom, but the resident was still injured as a result of the restraint. Does the plaintiff have any chance of proving that the defendant is nevertheless guilty of violating the common law duty of care?

Yes, if she can make a compelling argument that nursing homes in the area failed to establish a high enough duty of care. The plaintiff's job is to convince the judge that local custom condones substandard care, and that the defendant facility should be found liable for not knowing that its residents were inadequately protected.

The standard of care to which a nursing home will be held is always a case-by-case determination. A facility that is caring for a resident with known mental and physical limitations will be held to a higher standard of care than a facility that is treating a healthier and more self-sufficient resident. As the patient's capacity for self-care drops, the facility's duty of care rises.

Say two residents are injured while wandering away from the facility unattended. One patient was known by the facility to be a wanderer, while the other had always stayed in his room. The facility would be more likely to be found liable in connection with the known wanderer's injuries than those sustained by the homebody.

Despite the availability of claims for negligence, relatively few lawsuits are actually brought against nursing homes. There are a few explanations for this phenomenon.

First, the typical plaintiff encounters some logistical problems, not the least of which is finding a lawyer willing to take the case. Elderly plaintiffs are at risk of dying before the case is tried or settled. While not every lawsuit dies with the plaintiff, some do. Many lawyers are reluctant to invest their time and money in a case that may never result in a verdict or settlement.

The two primary predictors of whether a cause of action will survive the plaintiff's death are the nature of the action itself and who, if anyone, survives the plaintiff. Actions that are deemed purely personal do not survive the plaintiff's death. An action is also more likely to be dismissed upon the plaintiff's death if the patient is not survived by a spouse, child, parent, sibling, or other close family member.

In the context of suits against nursing facilities, the application of these predictors often works to the plaintiff's detriment. Where the acts of negligence or abuse are most egregious and result in the plaintiff's death, the offending facility is most likely to escape civil liability. All too often, the victim is not survived by a close relative. Many older people live in a nursing facility precisely because they have no close living relatives.

Lawyers who represent plaintiffs against nursing facilities also have some ominous legal obstacles to overcome. Their client may suffer memory or communication problems that make her a bad witness. Potential witnesses may include nursing home employees and other residents of the facility who are unwilling or unable to testify. Employees may withhold information about the facility's wrongdoing out of fear of reprisal, and the other nursing home residents may suffer sensory impairments of their own.

Where reliable witnesses are scarce, the lawyer must often rely on matters of public record to make their case. They hope and pray that annual inspection reports, reports of complaints, and certified financial statements will document substandard conditions in the facility. Unfortunately, documentary proof is rarely as compelling as the oral testimony of a live witness.

There are other evidentiary problems as well. The plaintiff must prove that the facility's failure to meet the standard of care was the direct cause of the plaintiff's injury. Without such proof of causation, the facility escapes liability.

In the run-of-the-mill negligence case, expert testimony establishes the causal link between the defendant's wrongdoing and the plaintiff's injuries. However, even experts in geriatric medicine often cannot definitively identify the cause of an elderly patient's decline. Was it the direct result of the defendant's wrongdoing, or an unavoidable consequence of the patient's advanced age or a preexisting medical condition? The distinction is often a difficult one to make with any degree of medical certainty.

A final problem encountered by nursing home plaintiffs relates to the assessment of damages. In most personal injury actions, damages are based on the victim's lost earning capacity, predicted life expectancy, number of dependents, and degree of pain and suffering. (See chapter 1.) Since nursing home residents have limited earning capacity, no dependents, and a short life expectancy, the potential for damages has traditionally been small. A small potential for damages means a small pool of available lawyers.

This is changing. Thanks in large part to the high standards set by the Nursing

Home Reform Law, increasing numbers of cases involving nursing home residents are resulting in six- and seven-figure verdicts and settlements. These large awards have been made to residents who were improperly assessed, illegally restrained, not provided with an individualized plan of care, or injured as a result of inadequate nursing home staffing.

In some jurisdictions, residents who are fortunate enough to get a generous award of damages do not derive any real benefit from their victory. Their receipt of the award causes their income and resources to rise so substantially that they become ineligible for public medical assistance (Medicaid), which is available only to people who can demonstrate financial need. Once ineligible for Medicaid, they must start paying for their nursing home care with private funds. In no time at all, their award is depleted on the exorbitant cost of private nursing home care, and they must reapply for Medicaid. They are back to square one; on Medicaid, with no money in the bank, and nothing to leave their heirs. The money paid by the nursing home as damages has been returned to the home as fees.

Some states protect the recoveries of nursing home residents by making the award exempt for Medicaid purposes. Other states allow the resident to invest the award in exempt assets, such as the family home. There are also some states that will allow the resident to use part of the award to pay a caregiving relative for his or her services.

CONTRACT LAW

The first part of this chapter reviewed the reform law requirement that federally certified nursing facilities must conform to a variety of standards in order to maintain their Medicare and Medicaid certification. These standards may be enforceable under state contract law (in addition to any implied private right of action that may be available under the reform law—see page 119).

Certified facilities sign a contract with the federal government (a "provider contract"). In return for the privilege of receiving Medicare and Medicaid reimbursement, these facilities agree to conform to the requirements of the reform law. Nursing home residents, though not parties to the provider contract, benefit from the agreement. As such, they are called "third party beneficiaries" of the provider contract.

Contract law gives third party beneficiaries the right to enforce contracts that affect their lives, even if they are not parties to the contract. A nursing home resident, in other words, can bring a breach of contract action against a nursing home for failing to meet its contractual obligations to comply with the reform law.[112]

Contract law protects the rights of nursing home residents in another way as well. As part of the nursing home admissions process, every incoming resident (or representative) is asked to sign an admissions agreement. This agreement, to which the resident *is* a party, also provides bases for breach of contract actions.

One breach of contract action based on the admissions agreement is premised on the reform law, even though the reform law itself is not contained in the text of the admissions agreement. Admissions agreements prepared by Medicare- and Medicaid-certified facilities implicitly incorporate the protections of the reform law. Incoming residents who sign the admissions agreements can (at least arguably) redress violations of the reform law by suing the facility for breach of contract.

Other contractual causes of action based on the admissions agreement have nothing to do with the reform law. They derive from the express provisions of the agreement itself.

Take, for example, admissions agreement provisions that relate to the payment of the nursing home bill. Contractual provisions concerning *who* pays the bills, *how much* they pay, and *when* they pay are near and dear to the heart of every nursing home. Nursing facilities operate in dread of having to "carry" a non-paying, or low-paying, resident.

Certain contractual payment provisions are now illegal because they discriminate against Medicare and Medicaid recipients. The nursing home cannot, for example, require the incoming resident to pay for her care privately for a stated period of time (so-called private-pay duration-of-stay provisions), or require the applicant to give assurances that he or she is not currently eligible for Medicaid, or require another individual, such as a family member, to co-sign the contract and assume personal financial responsibility for the resident's nursing home bill (so-called third-party guarantor provisions), or solicit contributions as a condition of admitting the applicant to the home.

Despite these beneficial restrictions on admissions contracts, the nursing home industry has found ways to comply with the letter of the law while arguably violating the spirit of the law. Take, for example, the common practice among nursing homes of requesting extensive financial documentation from incoming residents.

Advocates have argued for years that such an inquiry into an applicant's net worth eviscerates the intended protection of the law. It may be well and good that the applicant does not have to provide any express assurances about his or her Medicaid eligibility, but what good is this protection if the nursing home knows everything about the applicant's finances anyway? The nursing home knows how long the resident will be paying for her care privately by reviewing her net worth statement.

The legal merit of such an argument is debatable. What is not debatable, however, is the lengths to which a family will go in order to secure a desirable nursing home placement for a loved one. When admissions personnel at the nursing facility ask for the applicant's bank statements, most families turn over the statements. Nursing home beds are in short supply in many areas of the country, and few applicants for admission want to explore the outer reaches of their legal rights.

The practical protection of the prohibition against soliciting contributions from Medicaid applicants and persons related to the applicant is likewise questionable. Although a home may not break the law by making the applicant's admission conditional on the offer of a contribution, the families of Medicaid recipients may feel pressure to offer a contribution in the hopes of securing an elusive Medicaid-certified bed. The voluntariness of such a contribution is questionable.

What is the family's legal position when a "voluntary" contribution clearly facilitates the applicant's admission to the facility? Is there a basis for a lawsuit? Probably. Should the family sue? Arguably not. The risk of provoking the nursing facility into taking retaliatory action against the institutionalized loved one,[113] and the expense and hassle of a lawsuit, would discourage even the most principled families from suing.

The legal protection against third-party guarantor provisions also has its limits. The protection does not apply to individuals who have legal access to the applicant's income or resources. For example, a child who has been granted power of attorney can be legally required to use the parent's income and resources to pay the nursing home bill if the parent is admitted to the facility. Similarly, a court-appointed conservator or guardian of the resident's estate can be required to sign a contract promising to use the resident's own funds to pay the resident's nursing home bill.

If you are an attorney-in-fact appointed in a power of attorney or a court-appointed fiduciary, you want to be sure that you do not inadvertently become personally liable for the resident's nursing home bill. The best way to protect your interests is to always sign in your representative capacity. Sign your name followed by "as [insert resident's name]'s representative." Avoid signing your name without reference to the resident.

Another important set of provisions in the admissions agreement pertains to the goods and services the resident is entitled to receive while institutionalized in the nursing facility. A good admissions agreement spells out what is, and is not, included in the facility's per diem rate. A May 1995 study of California nursing homes found that 66.2 percent failed to list items and services not included in the basic daily rate.

The typical problem that arises in connection with the contractual description of covered goods and services is vagueness. Many contracts use general terms to describe covered items, such as "nursing and personal care sufficient to meet the resident's health, safety, and comfort needs." What does this mean? Should professional hairdressing services be provided at no extra cost to a resident who has had her hair professionally styled for her entire adult life? The answer is not always clear.

When a dispute arises over a facility's interpretation of the covered services portion of the contract, the resident is in a strong legal position. A well-settled legal principle provides that ambiguous contractual provisions should be construed *against* the party that drew up the agreement—in this case, the nursing facility.

Most courts, in applying this legal principle to a nursing home admissions agreement, would interpret any ambiguous coverage provisions in favor of the resident. The courts would recognize that the nursing home, as the drafter of the agreement, was better positioned to include provisions for its own benefit. Also, most courts would bend over backwards to protect the interests of the unsophisticated resident against the savvy nursing home administrator.

When the resident is covered by Medicare or Medicaid, the rules and regulations that govern those programs determine what items and services are and are not included within the per diem rate.

Often unbeknownst to them, residents and representatives who sign admissions agreements relinquish important legal rights. The agreements can include waivers of liability for property damage and, with somewhat less frequency, waivers for personal injury.

Typical waiver clauses read as follows:

[property damage]
The facility shall not be responsible for property damage, loss, or theft of any money, valuables, or personal effects brought into the facility by the resident or the resident's visitors unless said property is delivered to the custody of the facility's business office for safe keeping, and for which a receipt will be issued.

[personal injury]
The facility shall not be responsible for personal injuries caused to the resident by other patients in the facility, facility staff, or by independent contractors, and shall not be responsible for injuries that occur outside the facility, such as on a field trip.

The waiver concerning property damage or loss comes perilously close to violating the provisions of the Nursing Home Reform Law that protect the rights of residents to "retain and use [their] personal possessions and clothing as space permits." Residents who have no protection against the wrongful destruction or misappropriation of their property are unlikely to feel free to enjoy the full benefit of this statutory protection. The provision may well be unenforceable.

Waivers of responsibility for personal injury are almost certainly unenforceable. Though not exactly illegal, they fly in the face of the reform law mandate to nursing facilities to care for residents "in an environment that will promote maintenance or enhancement of the quality of life of each resident." They have also been found to be void as a matter of public policy in many jurisdictions.

Any nursing home agreement that includes language expanding the allowed circumstances for involuntary transfer and discharge should set off an alarm. Almost 92 percent of California nursing homes include illegal bases for transfer in their admissions agreement, according to a study of sixty-five randomly selected facilities. As already discussed, the law limits the permissible bases for transfer and discharge (see page 133).

Some facilities attempt to circumvent these legal restrictions by reserving to the facility the right to terminate the resident's contract upon a showing of intemperance, immorality, incompetency, cruelty, mental derangement, and/or the willful violation of laws, regulations, or rules. These provisions are unenforceable as a matter of law.

Other facilities provide that the resident's failure "to accept and pay for special nursing care when deemed necessary and proper by the home" is grounds for involuntary transfer or discharge. Once again, this provision is illegal. The refusal of nursing care is *not* one of the statutory bases for transfer or discharge. Furthermore, every resident's right to refuse medical and nursing treatment is protected by the statutory bill of rights and the U.S. Constitution (see chapter 6).

A related provision found in some admissions agreements concerns the movement of residents from one room to another within the same facility. The facility may reserve in the contract the discretion to change the resident's accommodations "in order to maintain efficiency and accord."

Federal law does not address transfers within the same facility ("intrafacility transfers") to the same extent as it regulates transfers to another facility ("interfacility transfers"). In fact, the federal reform law only requires the facility to provide notice to the resident before changing the resident's room or roommate. Some states have taken greater initiative in regulating intrafacility transfers.

The federal government's failure to protect nursing home residents from being indiscriminately moved from room to room within the same facility is unfortunate. Nursing home administrators are free to move residents around in the interest of operational efficiency, while the psychological trauma of being moved to a different wing of the same nursing home can be as devastating to a confused resident as an outside transfer (see page 133.) There is little residents can do when faced with an unwanted intrafacility relocation except research state-specific restrictions and procedural protections.

Nursing homes that have included deceptive or misleading provisions in their admissions agreement have been ordered to pay damages for violating consumer protection laws.[114] Misleading contractual provisions may give rise to other causes of action as well. If the offending facility belongs to an interstate chain, remedies may be available under antitrust law and Federal Trade Commission (FTC) rules. Where application of the disputed contractual provisions has a discriminatory impact on residents, a claim may be available under the Civil Rights Act and/or the Rehabilitation Act of 1973.

Suing a nursing home for breach of contract offers plaintiffs an important benefit—a longer statute of limitations. The statutue of limitations is the period of time within which a plaintiff must commence a lawsuit. The statute of limitations for contract actions can be considerably longer than the statute of limitations for negligence actions.

RESOURCES

For additional information about the rights of nursing home residents, call or write the following advocacy organizations:

Alzheimer's Association
1319 F Street, NW, Suite 710
Washington, D.C. 20004
202-393-7737

If you request the booklet Alzheimer Special Care in Nursing Homes: Is it Really Special? *you will be billed $5.*

AARP Fulfillment (EE0888)
601 E Street, NW
Washington, D.C. 20049
1-800-424-3410 (membership information)

The American Association of Retired Persons (AARP) also provides information on long-term nursing facilities. To order a free copy of Nursing Home Life: A Guide for Residents and Families, *request stock number D13063. For a slightly more technical discussion of the rights of nursing home residents, AARP's Legal Counsel for the Elderly makes available to the public a 245-page book entitled* A Practical Guide to Nursing Home Advocacy *(stock number D13878). The book can be ordered by sending $29.95 (AARP members) or $39.95 (nonmembers) plus $1.50 shipping and handling to Legal Counsel for the Elderly, P.O. Box 96474, Washington, D.C. 20090-6474.*

CAREsource Program Development, Inc.
500 Seattle Tower
1218 Third Avenue
Seattle, WA 98101-3021
206-625-9128

CAREsource has published a sixteen-page booklet entitled A Matter of Rights *that covers the rights of nursing home patients. The booklet is available in English, Spanish, Chinese, large-print type, and braille. The booklet costs $1.55 ($1.95 for large-print type and $15 for hardbound braille book). You can send payment or ask to be billed.*

Federation of Protestant Welfare Agency
Division on Aging
281 Park Avenue South
New York, NY 10010
212-777-4800

You can request the free manual How to Establish a Residential Council.

Friends and Relatives of the Institutionalized Aged (FRIA)

11 John Street, Suite 601
New York, NY 10038
212-732-4455

FRIA makes available to the public free booklets on food, mobility, overmedication, pressure sores, and restraints.

The National Citizens' Coalition for Nursing Home Reform (NCCNHR)

1424 16th Street, NW, Suite 202
Washington, D.C. 20036-2211
202-332-2275

NCCNHR has an extensive list of publications covering various aspects of nursing home patient rights. Contact the coalition to request a publication list. For a fee of $2 (nursing home resident), $10 (if sixty-five or over), or $40 (all others), you can become a member of NCCNHR. As a member you will receive a free subscription to the bimonthly newsletter (Quality Care Advocate), *a 20 percent discount on publications, and a discount registration fee for NCCNHR's annual meeting.*

The National Council of Senior Citizens

Nursing Home Information Service
National Senior Citizens Education and Research Center, Inc.
1331 F Street, NW
Washington, D.C. 22004-1171
202-347-8800

The Nursing Home Information Services is an information and referral center for consumers of long-term care and their representatives. The service provides information on nursing homes, including a free guide on how to select a nursing home.

SIX

Your Right of Medical Decision Making

True or False?

Your husband, already in the late stages of dementia, suffers a major stroke. He lapses into a coma and later develops pneumonia. His doctors advise you that they plan to start him on a course of antibiotics. You have a right to instruct the doctors to use medications only as needed to control your husband's pain, not to aggressively treat the pneumonia.

True or False?

In anticipation of the cross-country trip you and your husband plan to take from your home state of Florida to the golden coast of California, you sign a living will in accordance with Florida law. You become incapacitated somewhere in the middle of the country. The Midwest doctors are legally bound by your Florida directive

The short answer to both of these questions is "possibly false."
First, your legal authority to make health care choices for your husband, or anyone else, depends on the relevant state law. Second, state law controls medical directives, so a directive that is legally binding in one state may not bind doctors practicing medicine in a different state.

146

The subject of this chapter is medical decision making. Medical decisions include choices about whether you receive treatment, where you receive treatment, and the types of treatment you receive. Will you be treated at home or in a hospital? With radiation or chemotherapy? Sustained on life support or allowed to die?

This chapter addresses medical decision making while you are competent and after the onset of incapacity. It explores the scope of your right to make your own health care choices while you are competent, and the rights of others to make medical decisions on your behalf if you become incompetent to make those decisions for yourself.

Medical decision making is the raison d'être of the Right to Die movement. The movement's purpose is to preserve and protect the right of every competent adult to continue controlling his or her medical care after the onset of incapacity.

A strong argument can be made for renaming the Right to Die movement. Medical decision making entails far more than deciding whether or not to die. When you get sick, a myriad of questions arise about every aspect of your care. Which medical facility is best equipped to treat you? Should your condition be treated aggressively at the outset, or is a wait-and-see approach more advisable? How should the risks and benefits of alternative modes of treatment be balanced? Perhaps a more appropriate name for the movement is the Right of Medical Self-Determination, the Right to Certainty about Treatment, the Right to Relieve Loved Ones of the Burden of Health Care Decision Making, or the Right to Avoid the Economic Burden of Unnecessary Care. At the very least, these alternative appellations are less morbid. At best, they are more accurate.

As long as you are competent to make decisions about your care, these decisions are yours to make. Exclusively. No one can interfere with your health care decisions, even if your decisions differ from the choices your friends, family, or physicians would make.

Your right to control your medical care is firmly entrenched in the U.S. Constitution. Over 100 years ago, the Supreme Court decided that the constitutional right of privacy protected the right of each competent individual to determine what shall happen to his or her body.

The following examples demonstrate the reach of a competent patient's exclusive medical decision-making authority.

T.S., a seventy-five-year-old widower, had a long history of diabetes. When his doctors diagnosed the black patch on the bottom of his foot as gangrene, they recommended amputation. T.S. refused to consent to the procedure, even though he knew that the gangrene would probably spread and cause his death. Since the doctors had no reason to question T.S.'s mental capacity, they could not legally perform the amputation. T.S. died shortly thereafter.

A.J. was only fifty-five years old, but he was dependent on a ventilator. Amyotrophic lateral sclerosis (ALS, or Lou Gehrig's disease) had left him unable to breathe on his own. A.J. requested that he be removed from the ventilator and allowed to die. When his family and doctors refused to accede to his wishes, A.J. sued the hospital. He argued that the facility was violating his constitutional right of privacy by treating him against his will. The judge who heard the matter determined that A.J. had full decision-making capacity, and ordered the removal of the respirator.

Sally was the mother of two young children. When she was diagnosed with cancer, the doctors recommended a blood transfusion. She was told that she would die within five years if she did not undergo the procedure. Sally refused to consent to the transfusion. Since Sally's capacity to make decisions about her care was never in question, no one, not even Sally's husband, could force Sally to undergo the recommended treatment.

As these examples make clear, adult patients with decision-making capacity have complete and absolute control over their care.

But what about adult patients who have lost the capacity to make reasoned decisions about their own treatment? Decisions must still be made about their care, but by whom?

The first section of this chapter explores decision-making capacity. When is a patient capable or incapable of making decisions about his or her medical treatment? The second section covers medical decision making on behalf of incapacitated patients, specifically through the use of advance medical directives and do-not-resuscitate orders. The chapter concludes with a look at state surrogate decision-making laws and relevant federal legislation.

DECISION-MAKING CAPACITY

Dottie, a seventy-five-year-old widow, was diagnosed with throat cancer eight years ago. When she was told that the cancer had spread, she consented to undergo exploratory surgery. Dottie would not, however, consent to any surgery that would leave her unable to chew and swallow food on her own, even if such surgery was necessary to save her life.

Dottie's family, friends, and physicians thought she was "crazy" for refusing to consent to the life-saving surgery. They petitioned the court to force Dottie to undergo whatever surgery was necessary to save her life.

The judge who was asked to decide this case had to determine whether Dottie had decision-making capacity. Did she have the ability to understand the nature of the treatment options presented, appreciate the consequences of the various options, then make and communicate a reasoned choice?

To help him answer these questions, the judge heard evidence from a psychiatrist who examined Dottie. The judge learned that Dottie's short-term memory was not good, and she had fleeting periods of confusion. The psychiatrist testified that on a mental status exam Dottie could not remember lists of words and numbers, and could not count backward from one hundred by sevens. She did not know her age, and could not remember the president's name. She also failed to respond to some of the psychiatrist's questions, although her doctor testified that her hearing was not good and she might not have heard every question.

The judge also heard the testimony of Dottie's clergy, relatives, and friends. These witnesses conceded that Dottie had always been one to question doctors, resist taking prescription drugs, and leave the hospital against medical advice. She treasured her independence, and repeatedly declined invitations to move into the spare bedroom in her daughter's house.

Finally, the judge questioned Dottie. In her testimony, Dottie expressed an understanding that the doctors might have to surgically remove part of her throat and that she would likely die within weeks if the surgery was not performed. She clearly stated that she would rather die than be unable to eat "normally."

The judge decided that Dottie had the capacity to decide to forgo the disfiguring surgery. No apparent link existed between Dottie's memory problems and confusion and her ability to understand the nature and significance of her treatment decision. Furthermore, her decision appeared to be well reasoned.

A patient's well-reasoned decision must be upheld, even if the decision is not entirely reasonable. A reasoned decision, unlike a reasonable decision, may be utterly irrational to everyone other than the decision-maker. The judge knew Dottie's decision to refuse the surgery was well reasoned because it was consistent with her goals, values, and previously expressed wishes.

MEDICAL DECISION-MAKING AFTER INCAPACITY

What if the judge had determined that Dottie lacked the mental capacity to make reasoned decisions about her care? Then who would have made the decision about the surgery? Certainly not Dottie . . . unless, perhaps, Dottie had prepared an advance medical directive before she became incapacitated.

Broadly stated, an advance medical directive is a document that expresses an individual's wishes about what should happen in the event the individual becomes incapable of making medical treatment decisions for him- or herself. The discussion that follows examines the constitutional foundation for medical directives, state laws on medical directives, types of advance directives, and problems with advance directives.

MEDICAL DIRECTIVES AND OUR CONSTITUTIONAL RIGHTS

The Supreme Court made the medical directive a potent protector of patient rights in 1990 when it decided the case of Nancy Cruzan. The Cruzan case involved a twenty-five-year-old woman who lapsed into a persistent vegetative state (coma) following an automobile accident. Ms. Cruzan could breathe on her own, but appeared to lack all cognitive function and could not feed herself.

After four years of being sustained through a tube in her stomach, Nancy's parents requested the termination of the tube feedings. They were convinced that Nancy would never regain consciousness. They also believed that Nancy would have requested the termination of the tube feedings herself if she had the capacity to make and communicate that decision.

When the hospital refused to honor the Cruzans' request, a lawsuit ensued.

The Missouri court ruled on appeal that Nancy's feedings could not be terminated. The court found that Nancy's family had failed to submit "clear and convincing" evidence that Nancy would have wanted the feeding tube removed. The only evidence of Nancy's wishes was a passing comment Nancy had made to a roommate about not wanting to "live as a vegetable."

The court determined Nancy's aside to her roommate was not sufficiently reliable evidence of her health care wishes.

The Cruzans appealed the court's decision to the U.S. Supreme Court. In its decision, the High Court made the following points: First, competent patients have the right to refuse unwanted medical treatment. Second, incompetent patients have the right to have their treatment wishes carried out by another person. Third, states can constitutionally require a high degree of proof of a patient's health care wishes to ensure that decisions made on behalf of incompetent patients accurately reflect the patient's personal preferences.[115]

Applying these three principles to the facts of the Cruzan case, the issue became whether Missouri's requirement of clear and convincing evidence imposed an unconstitutionally high burden of proof on the surrogate decision-maker for an incompetent patient. The Supreme Court ruled that the standard passed constitutional muster. Unless and until Nancy Cruzan's parents could present clear and convincing evidence that their daughter would have wanted the feeding tube removed, they could not make that decision on Nancy's behalf.

Seven years later, the Cruzan family was finally able to present the court with clear and convincing evidence of Nancy's health care wishes. Colleagues who had worked with Nancy came forward to testify that Nancy had repeatedly stated that she would not want to be kept alive on a machine.[116] The court agreed that there was finally sufficient proof that Nancy would not have wanted to be maintained in a vegetative state, and authorized the removal of Nancy's feeding tube. Nancy died ten days later.

After the Cruzan case, there is no longer any question that an incompetent patient's health care wishes must be respected *if* there is adequate proof of what those wishes are. It is now up to the states to define what constitutes adequate proof of an incompetent patient's health care wishes. Adequate proof may be clear and convincing evidence of the patient's wishes, a very high standard of proof, or some lesser degree of proof, like a preponderance of the evidence.

Both oral and written statements can be used to prove an incompetent patient's treatment preferences. Oral statements are, however, inherently less reliable than written statements. Accordingly, the best way to leave proof of your health care wishes is to put those wishes in writing. An advance directive is a written statement of your health care wishes.

Probably the greatest motivation for preparing an advance directive is concern for your loved ones. When you communicate your treatment preferences in advance, you lighten the decision-making burden that would otherwise fall on the shoulders of concerned friends and family.

An advance directive gives your closest kin a written statement from you to rely on when making difficult choices on your behalf. The directive can relieve the decision-makers of the guilt associated with declining treatments, and head off disagreements among family members.

One can only theorize as to why only 15 to 20 percent of Americans have signed an advance directive. Fear probably has a lot to do with it.

There may be fear that doctors will use the advance directive to withhold needed treatment. Studies finding a correlation between economic class and the willingness to sign a directive lend credence to the theory that many people do not sign directives out of fear that doctors might use the directive to the patient's detriment.

People in the middle and upper-middle classes are more likely to sign a directive than those in the lower economic classes. Is it coincidence that wealthy people are also more likely to have a long-standing relationship with a trusted physician? Low-income patients who often lack a primary care physician do have greater reason to worry that a directive could be used to wrongfully withhold treatment.

Fear of death also provides a strong disincentive to preparing an advance directive. You cannot sign a medical directive without confronting your mortality. Death does not win first place on most people's top ten list of favorite topics of conversation, for good reason. Why discuss the impending cessation of conscious existence when you could talk about a tasty dish of food or a spectacular sunset? Nevertheless, the importance of openly discussing such disturbing subjects as terminal illness, irreversible comas, and imminent death cannot be overstated.

Discussing issues of life and death helps you formulate your own health care wishes. You cannot communicate your treatment preferences to others if you have not discovered them yourself. Furthermore, even if you never actually sign a medical directive, the discussions themselves will provide important proof of your health care wishes and may influence the care you receive if you are ever incapacitated.

Ironically, the very ill and elderly, for whom death is a reality, more readily broach the subject of their own mortality than the young and healthy, for whom death is more remote. In many cases, friends and relatives resist a dying person's efforts to speak openly and frankly about what lies ahead.

When the patient speaks of being ready to die, loved ones may insist that the patient is doing fine. The patient's efforts to discuss his or her declining health may be dismissed with such reassuring comments as, "Don't be silly. You're not dying."

Though understandable, this is an unfortunate state of affairs. Loved ones that mean to be encouraging and supportive may actually be cheating those close to death of the opportunity to confront and resolve their fears and regrets.

People who are approaching death should be encouraged to talk about the dying process. The subject of death can be broached in any number of ways. The best approach depends on the personalities of the parties involved. Here are some suggestions:

➤ Be available. Simply ask the patient if there is anything she would like to talk about.

➤ Be up-front. Ask the patient if she has been thinking about her impending death. Find out if there is anything she would like to discuss with you.

➤ Be curious. Tell the patient you would like to learn more about what she is going through. What does she think about? What frightens her the most?

If you find yourself reluctant to raise the subject of death, remember this: Bereavement counselors find that one of the greatest sources of anger in survivors is uncertainty about whether the deceased was treated as he or she would have wanted.

By speaking about matters of death in advance, you can play a positive role in the patient's dying process. You can make sure your loved one's treatment preferences are respected. Your knowledge that everything connected with your loved one's passing was as your loved one wanted it to be may become a great source of comfort to you later.

Death is rarely an instantaneous occurrence. More often it is a process fraught with difficult decisions that must be made by someone. Why shouldn't the someone be the person who is dying?

The right of competent adults to control their medical care after the onset of incapacity was publicized recently by the very public deaths of Richard Nixon and Jacqueline Kennedy Onassis. Each of these prominent figures used an advance directive to forgo medical treatment that might have prolonged his or her life.

Mrs. Onassis prepared a living will in February 1994 after she began receiving treatment for lymphoma. When she was told in April 1994 that the cancer had spread to her brain and liver, she chose to go home to die. The former president was also allowed to die in accordance with his previously expressed wishes, four days after suffering a debilitating stroke. After Mr. Nixon's death on April 22, 1994, Choice in Dying, a non-profit organization that distributes free advance directive forms (see page 170), reported a surge in requests for information about living wills—from about 100 a day to 2,000 a day. At least for the short term, people were attracted by the notion of retaining control over their treatment decisions.

Although most patients use advance directives to decline medical treatment, directives are equally effective in communicating an incompetent patient's wish to receive the benefit of all life-sustaining medical treatment, even if there is no possibility of recovery.

A recent Massachusetts case forced a court to address a situation where a seventy-one-year-old woman with irreversible brain damage had left verbal instructions with her daughter that everything medically possible should be done in the event the mother became incompetent. When the daughter communicated these treatment preferences to the doctors and hospital responsible for her mother's care, the providers said they were unwilling to honor the patient's wishes on the grounds that additional medical care would be futile. In apparently the first lawsuit to test whether doctors must provide futile medical treatment in accordance with an incompetent patient's previously expressed health care wishes, the court sided with the doctors.

The chairman of the ethics committee at New England Medical Center responded to the court's decision by stating that conflicts between doctors wanting to withhold futile care and families wanting to prolong treatment arise virtually every week. Before the decision was rendered, doctors almost always provided the care, believing it was their legal obligation to do so.[117] Whether they will continue to do so remains to be seen.

STATE LAWS ON ADVANCE DIRECTIVES

As you now know, every spoken and written expression of your health care wishes has legal effect if and when you become unable to make medical treatment decisions for yourself. However, each state can determine *how* much proof of an incompetent patient's health care wishes is enough proof to empower someone to make treatment decisions on that patient's behalf.

State legislatures across the country have passed laws that govern medical decision making on behalf of incompetent patients. Many of these laws specify a particular type of document that competent adults should use to memorialize their health care wishes. These documents are called advance medical directives.

An advance medical directive that conforms to state law constitutes sufficient proof of an incompetent patient's health care wishes *in that state*. Doctors licensed to practice medicine in the state are legally obligated to respect the patient's health care wishes as those wishes are expressed in the conforming advance directive. Providers that fail to honor the directive may face punitive action.

State laws on advance directives help you exercise your constitutional right to control your care. They tell you how to express your health care wishes while competent so those wishes will be binding on your providers if you become incompetent. A chart listing every state's law on advance directives, as well as sample directives, appears in appendix 10.

State laws on advance directives *do not limit* your constitutional right to receive care consistent with your prior verbal and written expressions of treatment preferences *even if those expressions do not conform to the state law. Every* prior expression of a health care preference still has legal effect. But prior expressions of health care preferences that do not conform to state law are not legally binding on medical providers.

Say you live in a state that has a law on advance directives. The law requires doctors to honor any written expression of a patient's health care wishes as long as the writing is notarized and witnessed. Say a resident puts his health care wishes in writing but neglects to get the statement notarized. The patient becomes incapacitated. What is the legal effect of the document?

The document still constitutes compelling evidence of the patient's health care wishes, even though it does not conform to the state law on advance directives. A court must decide, however, whether under state law the document constitutes *sufficient* evidence of the patient's health care wishes to control the patient's care after the onset of incapacity. The document, standing alone, will not be legally binding on doctors treating the incapacitated patient.

TYPES OF ADVANCE DIRECTIVES

Most state laws on advance directives authorize one of two types of medical directives; the living will (sometimes referred to as a "declaration" or "directive") or power of attorney for health care (sometimes referred to as a "health care proxy"). These two types of directives are discussed immediately below. The section closes with a quick look at do-not-resuscitate orders.

Living Will

A living will is an individual's statement of the treatments he or she does and does not want to receive in the event of a terminal illness or irreversible condition. Living wills come into play only if the individual is unable to make or communicate instructions about his or her care.

The typical living will statute includes the following provisions:

➤ Life-prolonging or life-sustaining treatments may be withheld or withdrawn from a patient who has prepared a document that complies with the formal requirements of the law. (Some states do not permit implementation of living wills on behalf of pregnant patients.)

➤ One or two physicians must certify in writing that the patient is terminally ill or, in some states, in a persistent vegetative state. Terminal illness is generally defined as an irreversible condition that will shortly lead to death. A persistent vegetative state is characterized by irregular cycles of sleeping, waking, and arousal, but without detectable cognition or awareness.

➤ Health care providers who withhold or withdraw life-prolonging treatment in good faith reliance on a living will are not subject to civil or criminal penalties.

➤ Refusal of life-prolonging treatment by a terminally ill patient does not constitute suicide for insurance or other purposes.

➤ Health care providers who, for religious or personal reasons, are unwilling to comply with the patient's instructions as set forth in a living will must transfer the patient to another provider who will honor the directive.

➤ Failure by a health care provider to follow a patient's valid directive or transfer the patient to another's care constitutes unprofessional conduct. In some states, noncompliance is a misdemeanor.

➤ Living wills must be signed in the presence of at least two adult witnesses. In some states one or both witnesses are prohibited from being a relative, a potential estate beneficiary, a legally responsible relative, or the patient's health care provider. Some states have special witness requirements for nursing home residents and hospital patients, require a notary, and/or require filing with a government office.

➤ Patients must notify their physicians that they have signed a living will, and then physicians must include a copy of the living will in the patient's medical record.

➤ A living will can always be revoked. Oral revocation is generally sufficient.

As a general matter, living wills can be used to terminate life-sustaining medical treatment. However, about half the states apply special restrictions to the withdrawal of tube-feedings and hydration. In these states, a living will cannot be relied on to terminate life-sustaining nutrition and hydration. All other types of life-sustaining medical treatment may be withdrawn pursuant to the patient's instructions as set forth in a living will.

According to a study published in the *Journal of the American Medical Association*, the exclusion of artificial feeding and hydration may actually increase the suffering of terminally ill patients. Starvation causes dehydration, which lessens consciousness, promotes sleepiness, and diminishes pain. The study also found that the terminally ill patients who asked not to be given food or liquids through tubes generally did not experience hunger when the artificial feedings were withdrawn.[118]

Most state living will statutes leave the drafting of the document to the individual. A minority of states require that living wills include certain statutory language. If you live in one of these states, you want your living will to include the precise text that appears in the state statute. You are permitted, however, to make changes and additions to the standard language. You should modify the form to reflect your personal and well-considered health care wishes. Never sign a preprinted "standard" directive without making sure the document reflects your own values and priorities.

A living will that is legally valid in one state may not meet the statutory requirements of another state. This lack of uniformity results in obvious practical difficulties.

As a resident of State A you sign a living will refusing any life-prolonging medical treatment in the event you are diagnosed with an irreversible coma. You suffer a stroke while in State B on business, and are not expected to emerge from the resulting coma. State B's law on living wills applies only in cases involving terminal illness. What effect, if any, will your living will have in State B?

It's difficult to say for sure. Some states give legal recognition to out-of-state advance directives that meet the requirements of the state in which the document was executed, while other states apply the law of the state in which the patient is receiving treatment. Still other states do not expressly address the issue one way or the other.

Ordinarily, in the absence of any controlling law, the requirements of the state where treatment occurs will prevail over those of the state where the document was signed. If the directive does not conform to the law in the treatment state, the providers in that state should still be encouraged to follow the directive as compelling evidence of the patient's wishes. The treating providers will not, however, be legally required to honor the directive if the directive does not conform to the technical requirements of their state law.

A living will is of no benefit if no one knows it exists. You can conscientiously give a copy of your living will to your primary physician, but if your physician is basking in the Tahitian sun when you lapse into a coma it will do you no good. To protect yourself, make several copies of your living will. (Copies have the same legal effect as the original.) Distribute the copies of the living will to the admissions personnel in your local hospitals, close friends and family members, and your clergy. Also, keep a copy of the directive in your purse or wallet, or a card stating the existence and location of the directive.

What if you prepare a living will in a state that does not have a living will statute? What is the legal effect, if any, of the directive?

The answer to this question will depend, to some extent, on state law. In New York, where there is no living will statute, a living will still has potent legal effect. The highest court in New York has found that a living will constitutes "clear and convincing evidence" of an incompetent patient's health care wishes. As such, a living will controls patient care after the onset of incapacity despite the absence of any state living will statute.[119]

Powers of Attorney for Health Care

You are probably already familiar with the use of powers of attorney for financial management. With a financial power of attorney, one individual (called a "principal") gives another individual (called an "agent") control over the principal's money and property.

People sign financial powers of attorney to enable others to sell property, pay bills, and change investments on their behalf. Without a financial power of attorney, no one has any legal authority over another person's assets.

Health care powers of attorney work on the same principle. An individual who signs a health care power of attorney authorizes an agent (or "proxy") to make health care decisions on the signer's behalf. The power of attorney becomes effective only if the signer becomes unable to make health care decisions for him- or herself. Without a health care power of attorney, no one has any legal authority to make health care decisions for another individual, not even a spouse or child (in the absence of state law to the contrary).

The use of powers of attorney in the area of medical decision making is still fairly new. In 1983, the President's Commission prepared a report approving the use of powers of attorney to appoint agents to make health care decisions. Today, laws specifically allowing the use of health care powers of attorney are on the books in about two-thirds of the states.

A health care power of attorney can be general or specific. General powers authorize agents to make any and all decisions on behalf of the principal, while specific powers limit the agent's authority to particular types of decisions or a particular time period. Health care powers rarely spell out the treatment choices that the agent is to make under specific circumstances. Occasionally, the power may include written instructions to guide the agent's decision making.

There are a few general rules to keep in mind when you sign a power of attorney for health care:

➤ Designate one or more successor agents. This is advisable in case your primary agent is unable or unwilling to serve.

➤ If you plan to use a standard power of attorney form (available for minimal cost at legal stationery stores), be sure your state does not have special requirements that apply specifically to powers of attorney for health care.

➤ Do not designate as an agent any doctor with responsibility for your care. Such a designation may violate state law. Prohibitions against the selection of a treating physician as an agent are intended to avoid situations where the physician/agent's medical judgment conflicts with his or her knowledge of the patient's health care wishes.

➤ Check state law before appointing a priest, rabbi, or any other agent who might be named in several other health care powers. In some states, an agent is permitted to represent only a specified number of principals.

➤ The health care power of attorney should be witnessed by two adults who are neither related to you nor responsible for your medical treatment and/or notarized. State laws have different execution requirements.

➤ Some states require the appointed agent to sign the power of attorney as well as the principal in order to indicate a willingness to serve.

➤ If you want to change your health care power of attorney, sign a new document. Try to recover and destroy all copies of the old power.

State laws on health care powers of attorney are not uniform. In a few states, agents appointed under a power of attorney cannot request the termination of artificial nutrition and hydration unless they are specifically given authority to make such decisions. In other states, the agent is not permitted to make decisions about life-sustaining medical treatment without specific written instructions from the principal, or actual knowledge of the patient's wishes regarding this type of care.

The most important rule of all when preparing a health care power of attorney is to discuss your health care wishes with your agent in advance of any medical crisis. Depending on the extent of authority you give your agent, the discussion should cover such issues as where you want to receive treatment, how you feel about entering a nursing home, your opinions about hospice care, and the circumstances under which you would consent to the use of feeding tubes and other life-sustaining treatment.

As with the living will, you should make several copies of the durable power of attorney. Give a copy to your primary and alternate agents, your doctor, local health care facilities, and close friends and family. You may also want to keep a copy of the power with you in your purse or wallet. Do not store your power of attorney in a safe-deposit box or any place that is not easily accessible to others.

Even if you live in a state that does not recognize health care powers of attorney by statute, your designation of an agent for health care decision making may still have legal effect. Just as living wills are recognized even in states that lack a living will statute, the appointment of an agent for medical decision making constitutes evidence of your health care wishes.

The agent named in your health care power may, for example, be consulted in connection with decisions that must be made about your care. You cannot be sure, however, that your health care providers will defer to your agent's instructions in the absence of a statutory mandate. Some states prohibit medical decision making by agents.

Certain individuals are unable or unwilling to prepare a health care power of attorney, even when allowed by state law. They may not want to burden anyone with the onerous responsibility of deciding whether they live or die. Or perhaps they don't have anyone to appoint as their health care agent. Their contemporaries are in poor health themselves, and family may live far away.

A living will provides individuals in this situation with an opportunity to leave clear evidence of their treatment preferences without involving another individual in decisions about their care. As already mentioned, living wills are compelling evidence of a patient's health care preferences even where the directive is not authorized by state law.

CHOOSING BETWEEN A LIVING WILL AND A HEALTH CARE AGENT

If you live in a state with a living will or health care power of attorney statute, you stand the best chance of having your health care wishes respected if you prepare a medical directive that conforms to the law in your state. That said, under certain circumstances it makes sense to execute both types of directives, even if one directive is not regulated by state law.

People who spend a lot of time outside their state of residence are often well advised to prepare both types of directives. If you have a living will that conforms to your state's law but you fall ill out-of-state, your health care power of attorney may come to your rescue. Every state recognizes financial powers of attorney, and some explicitly permit health care decision making by agents. Similarly, a living will constitutes good evidence of your health care wishes wherever your travels take you, even if your home state only recognizes health care powers of attorney by statute.

Other reasons you may want to prepare both types of documents have to do with the relative benefits and limitations of health care powers of attorney and living wills. Health care powers are generally more flexible, but they are also more burdensome on loved ones.

Health care powers of attorney are far more versatile than living wills. A living will only comes into play if you are diagnosed with a terminal illness or, in some states, a persistent vegetative state. If you suffer from an acute illness, such as a heart attack, or a chronic degenerative condition, such as Lou Gehrig's disease (or ALS), your living will may be irrelevant.

A general health care power of attorney, on the other hand, is relevant to almost any situation that entails medical decision making. Your health care agent can be authorized to review medical records and make decisions regarding amputation, dialysis, antibiotics, and a full range of other treatments on your behalf if you become incapacitated and suffer from a chronic and degenerative, but not terminal, illness.

A health care power also offers you the benefit of a living, breathing advocate. Unlike a living will, which is an easily ignored, inert piece of paper, the person you appoint in your power of attorney can take an active role in your care. Your agent can affirmatively hire and fire doctors, move you out of an unsatisfactory facility, and aggressively fight to overcome any resistance that is mounted to the implementation of your treatment preferences.

Along these same lines, a health care power of attorney also offers you the benefit of a thinking advocate. Your agent will be able to consider your doctor's recommendations in light of your previously expressed treatment preferences, weigh risks and benefits, and make a reasoned decision about the best course of care to pursue. A living will, in contrast, is based on a hypothetical set of circumstances that may bear no resemblance to the specific circumstances that exist at the time treatment decisions must be made on your behalf—that is, of course, assuming you write your living will without the benefit of a crystal ball.

Finally, a health care agent can serve an important function as interpreter. If you signed a living will that included a general statement about not wanting any treatments that only prolong the dying process, your agent could shed light on what you might have meant by such a statement. Would you have wanted life-prolonging medical treatment that gave you a one-in-three chance of recovering enough to return home for another six months? What about another three months? What about a one-in-ten chance of recovery? Your health care agent, presumably familiar with your values and wishes, would be in a better position than your doctors to interpret your intentions behind the ambiguous language of your living will.

We should note, however, a risk associated with preparing both types of directives. A conflict may arise between your wishes as expressed by your health care agent and your wishes as expressed in your living will.

Imagine, for example, that you have appointed your son as your health care agent in a power of attorney. You have also signed a living will stating that you do not want doctors to use heroic measures to prolong your life. When you can no longer make choices about your care, a decision must be made about trying a new experimental drug. Your son wants the doctors to start the treatment, but the doctors resist. They point to your living will, arguing that the new drug regimen would constitute a heroic measure.

This potential conflict can be easily avoided. Include in the living will a provision that "any conflicts should be resolved in favor of the agent appointed in my health care power of attorney." This provision will authorize your health care agent to interpret ambiguous provisions in your living will, and give your agent ultimate decision-making authority.

PREPARING AN ADVANCE DIRECTIVE

The first step in perparing an advance directive is to obtain sample directives that conform to the law in your state in addition to one or two other directives. Sample directives are usually available from local hospitals, state departments of health (see appendix 1), bar associations, state medical associations, and state or local offices on aging and legal services offices. You can also obtain a sample directive from the non-profit advocacy organization Choice in Dying (see resources at end of chapter).

Review the sample forms for your drafting options. Take pen in hand and modify the form that most closely reflects your wishes. The final document you produce should accurately convey your feelings about the appropriate and inappropriate use of medical interventions.

The next step is to discuss your health care preferences with your physician and close friends and family. If you are preparing a health care power of attorney or proxy, you must have such a discussion with the persons you appoint as your decision-making agents. In the course of the discussions, you may refine your thoughts about your treatment wishes. Modify your directive accordingly.

Finally, execute your directive in accordance with the technical requirements of the law in your state. Most states require two disinterested witnesses to sign the directive. Other states require a notary.

Although most people do not need an attorney to prepare an advance directive, your situation may be different. If you foresee the potential for conflict among family members, or if you have other special concerns, you should consult with an attorney who has special experience in elder law or estate planning.

PROBLEMS WITH ADVANCE DIRECTIVES

The biggest problem with advance directives is that not enough people have them. A 1993 study found only about one in ten respondents had a living will, although 90 percent favored the idea of an advance directive.

Another problem with medical directives is that too many doctors ignore them. Physicians in hospitals and nursing homes override medical directives in about 25 percent of the cases.[120] A November 1995 study reported in the *Journal of the American Medical Association* found that doctors often misunderstand or ignore the last wishes of dying patients. According to the researchers, nothing has changed in the twenty-five years that have passed since the birth of the right-to-die movement. Patients are suffering the same amount of pain at the end of life, and equal numbers of people are dying attached to machines.[121]

Sometimes doctors who are willing to honor the patient's instructions as set forth in a living will find themselves unable to discern the patient's true intent from the language in the document. Examples illustrating the problems that arise in interpreting living wills follows below:

➤ A patient whose living will specifies no life-sustaining treatments in the event of terminal illness develops pneumonia. The treatment for pneumonia is antibiotics. Although antibiotics are not really "life-sustaining," it is unclear whether the terminally ill cancer patient would want to undergo aggressive antibiotic treatment of the pneumonia.

➤ A nursing home resident becomes gravely ill after receiving the incorrect medication. Her living will states that she wishes to forgo all "heroic measures." Does this language mean the doctors should not give her the treatment she requires to recover from the effects of the incorrect medication?

➤ Would a patient who requests in his living will no antibiotics in the event of advanced irreversible dementia want to receive penicillin if infected with a painful skin condition?

As long as people cannot predict the future, these questions are bound to arise no matter how carefully the directive is drafted.

In other cases, doctors do not follow the patient's advance directive because the doctor is unaware that the directive exists. The patient may not have arranged for the directive to be included in his or her medical record, or the patient's loved ones may be too distraught to inform the providers about the patient's directive, or the nursing home may have transferred the patient to the hospital for treatment without transferring the patient's advance directive.

Finally, some doctors do not rely on a living will out of fear that they will be sued or prosecuted for their failure to prolong the patient's life. This fear of legal exposure persists despite the fact that no provider has ever been successfully sued or prosecuted for relying in good faith on an advance directive, according to a spokesman for the right-to-die advocacy group Choice in Dying. Many providers are under the incorrect assumption that they need a court order to carry out an advance directive.

Advance directives are legally binding on providers in the absence of a court order. In fact, a few courts have allowed lawsuits to proceed against doctors who decided to treat their patients in contravention of an advance directive.

While a lawsuit to enforce a directive may be an option, it is certainly not a desirable option. Lawsuits do not benefit patients who are left to live out a life of little or no quality after receiving treatment contrary to their stated instructions. When doctors put eighty-eight-year-old Dr. Perry Elfmont on oxygen and intravenous antibiotics after a suspected stroke, in direct violation of a statement in his living will that he did not want either type of intervention, his wife decided against suing the hospital. Instead, she wrote the hospital a letter expressing her dismay at how her husband's wishes had been violated.

Equally disconcerting is evidence that family members, who are usually called upon to interpret living wills and serve as health care agents, frequently fail to accurately predict the patient's health care wishes. One study found that family members who were asked whether the patient would want treatment under certain circumstances actually matched the patient's wishes only 70 percent of the time. The family members generally erred on the side of overtreatment.[122]

Some medical ethicists have another problem with living wills. They reject the underlying assumption that an individual's health care preferences remain the same after the onset of incapacity. They theorize, instead, that a healthy and competent individual's values and interests change when that individual becomes an incompetent patient.

These ethicists argue that incompetent patients have more limited interests and concerns than competent individuals. Treatments that appear to be distasteful and wasteful to competent individuals might be valued by these same individuals if they became incompetent patients. They argue further that competent individuals who refuse life-sustaining medical treatment in advance of incompetency may actually deprive their incompetent selves of the care they need and desire. Advocates of this theory cite in support of their arguments incompetent people who have been treated in contravention of their medical directive, and express appreciation for the care they received.

DO NOT RESUSCITATE ORDERS

Do-not-resuscitate (DNR) orders are a special type of advance medical directive. They apply only to decisions about whether or not to resuscitate a patient who has suffered cardiac or respiratory arrest. Every other type of medical treatment falls outside the scope of a DNR order.

With cardiac arrest (commonly known as a heart attack), the heart stops pumping. With respiratory arrest, breathing stops. Under either scenario, the patient cannot survive without resuscitation. The heart must be restarted or air must be pumped into the patient's lungs.

Resuscitation, even when successful, can come at a serious cost to the patient. Many patients who survive resuscitation efforts suffer extensive brain damage. In other cases, there is pain. Some patients experience anger or humiliation when they learn of the measures taken to prolong their life. A recent study found that most older adults, after learning that their chances of survival are only 10 to 17 percent, would prefer not to have cardiopulmonary resuscitation (CPR) following cardiac arrest.[123]

Where there is a state law authorizing a DNR order, the patient or the patient's representative can sign a document instructing the doctors to forgo all resuscitation efforts. Although the details of DNR legislation vary from state to state, most laws include the following provisions:

➤ In the absence of a DNR order, patients are presumed to consent to resuscitation efforts.

➤ Every adult is presumed capable of deciding to decline resuscitation. A physician is permitted to place a DNR order on the chart of a competent adult patient only after first obtaining the patient's consent. The patient's consent may not be required where there is evidence that discussion of the DNR order would result in the patient's immediate and severe injury, where a surrogate decision-maker has already been appointed, or where there is a relevant court order.

➤ Designated family members can consent to a DNR order on behalf of an incapacitated patient.

➤ DNR orders must be in writing and signed, dated, and witnessed. Oral DNR requests may be permitted under certain circumstances.

➤ Physicians treating patients with DNR orders must comply with the order or transfer the patient to another physician who will comply with the order.

➤ DNR orders must be reviewed periodically to see that the order is still appropriate in light of changes in the patient's medical condition.

A study reported in the *Journal of the American Medical Association* found that more than a third of resident doctors at Seattle hospitals followed patients' DNR orders, even though they believed that life-saving measures could have revived at least 5 percent of the patients. The study raised the important question of whether doctors should have absolute power to withhold resuscitation, even in light of the patients' wishes as expressed in a DNR request. In 12 percent of the cases, the doctors made the decision to withhold resuscitation without consulting the patient or the patient's representative.[124]

Some states have recently expanded their DNR laws to cover patients who are receiving care at home. Whereas DNR orders have been available to hospital and nursing home patients for some time, the new legislation enables patients being treated at home to decline resuscitation.

There is an obvious practical problem with enforcing DNR orders in the home care context. Unlike patients residing in a medical facility, patients living at home do not have a sign on their door, or file on their bed, to indicate their wishes regarding resuscitation.

New York has solved this implementation problem by providing home care patients with a bracelet when they are discharged from the hospital. The bracelet indicates that a DNR order has been signed. Emergency medical personnel in the state have been trained to respect the patient's wishes as expressed on the bracelet, except under limited circumstances.

SURROGATE DECISION-MAKING LAWS

Some states have in place a statutory scheme for appointing an alternative decision-maker for incapacitated patients who are incapable of making or communicating their own treatment choices. These so-called surrogate decision-making laws can exist instead of, or in addition to, the advance directive laws discussed in the previous section.

The following story is true.

When he was only twenty-one years old, ten days before his wedding, Joey Fiori was in a motorcycle accident. He sustained extensive brain damage. After intensive rehabilitation, Mr. Fiori could speak a few words and play cards.

Five years after the accident, a doctor at the Veterans Administration Hospital in Philadelphia gave Mr. Fiori the wrong medication. Mr. Fiori entered a vegetative state, unable to think, feel, speak, see, hear, smell, move, or swallow.

The federal government, acknowledging liability, began paying more than $150,000 a year for Mr. Fiori's care. Mr. Fiori's doctors said their patient could live for another twenty years in his condition. Joey Fiori's mother wanted her son's feeding tube removed.

Although Pennsylvania now has living will and health care power of attorney legislation, Mr. Fiori had not prepared an advance directive before he was injured more than twenty years ago. Mr. Fiori's mother was told by attorneys for the state that she could not have her son's life support removed unless she could present compelling evidence that he would have wanted the life support removed. Mrs. Fiori had no such proof of her young son's wishes; in all likelihood, Joey had probably not given his own death much thought.[125]

Joey Fiori slipped through cracks in the laws that govern the "right to die." He left neither an advance directive nor other evidence of his treatment preferences. Joey Fiori is not, of course, the only patient left in this predicament. His plight can befall any patient, especially a young patient, who loses capacity without leaving proof of his health care wishes.

Patients like Joey are protected by state surrogate decision-making laws. These laws provide an alternative decision-making procedure for patients who cannot make their own health care decisions and who have not adequately expressed their health care preferences in advance.

Two types of surrogate decision-making laws are family consent acts and guardianship (or conservatorship) laws. Each type of legislation is covered directly below.

FAMILY CONSENT ACTS

Family consent acts automatically vest decision-making authority in certain designated individuals ("surrogates"). The specifics of family consent laws vary from state to state.

Most family consent acts include provisions to the following effect:

➤ The patient is presumed to be capable of making health care decisions for him- or herself in the absence of a physician's certification to the contrary. Some states allow surrogate decision making only in cases involving terminal illness; other states accept a diagnosis of a permanent vegetative state.

➤ Surrogate decision-makers are to be appointed in the order listed in the statute. The common order of priority is court-appointed guardian, spouse, adult child, parent, and adult sibling. A close adult friend or relative who is familiar with the patient's health care wishes is usually last on the list, and appointed only if no guardian or family member is available.

➤ The scope of the surrogate's authority can include all medical decisions, with certain limits applying to decisions regarding life-sustaining medical treatment. Other states prohibit surrogates from making decisions regarding sterilization, abortion, and/or treatment of mental disorders. The surrogate must make medical decisions based on the patient's wishes, if known, or the patient's best interests.

➤ Decisions that must be made on behalf of patients who lack available surrogate decision-makers are generally left to one or more physicians, sometimes in consultation with an ethics review committee.

Even if your state does not have a family consent law, your loved ones may still be able to participate in decisions regarding your care if you become ill. Many hospitals and physicians informally rely on the preferences of family members in making treatment decisions. Especially when doctors and family unanimously agree on a course of care, the formal appointment of a surrogate decision-maker often becomes unnecessary. The lack of clear legal authority on the part of the family to make decisions on the patient's behalf may not prove insurmountable.

As mentioned in the introduction to this section, a family consent act can coexist with a medical directive statute. An example demonstrates how.

Mike lives in a state that has a family consent act and a living will act. While healthy, Mike signs a living will that conforms to state law. He falls off a scaffold and lapses into a coma. Under the family consent act his wife, Melanie, has legal authority to make decisions about Mike's care. In the event of a conflict, the living will would preempt Melanie's decision-making authority. Melanie would only have the authority to make decisions with respect to treatment choices that were not covered by Mike's validly executed directive.

GUARDIANSHIP AND CONSERVATORSHIP LAWS

Unlike living will laws, health care proxy statutes, and family consent acts, which an individual state may or may not have, each of the fifty states and the District of Columbia have some type of guardianship and/or conservatorship law on the books. Although the details of these laws are far from uniform, courts in every state of the nation have statutory authority to appoint an individual ("guardian" or "conservator") to act on behalf of another individual who is unable to act for him- or herself ("ward").

Guardianships and conservatorships. Conservatorships and guardianships. To the confusion of many, these terms are often used interchangeably.

For purposes of this discussion, both terms will be used to describe any proceeding whereby a court appoints a trustee to manage the property and/or person of an incapacitated individual. A property guardian has authority to make decisions regarding the ward's money and real estate, while a personal guardian has authority to decide where the ward will live, whom the ward will associate with, and what activities the ward will pursue. The scope of permissible decision-making authority is broad, and touches on the ward's most fundamental liberties.

Guardianship and conservatorship laws manifest each state's interest in caring for residents who are either unwilling or unable to care for themselves. This authority derives in part from the old common-law doctrine of *parens patriae*. This benevolent doctrine empowers state governments to act as a parent to residents in need of assistance.

Although each state has its own procedures and standards, most guardianship/ conservatorship proceedings share the following features:

➤ A guardian can be appointed only if the proposed ward meets the definition of an "incapacitated person." Although this definition varies from state to state, most jurisdictions have adopted language similar to that which appears in the Uniform Probate Code (UPC). The UPC, a model for guardianship legislation nationwide, defines an incapacitated person as one "who is impaired by reason of mental illness, mental deficiency, physical illness or disability, advanced age, chronic use of drugs, chronic intoxication, or other cause (except minority) to the extent of lacking sufficient understanding or capacity to make or communicate responsible decisions."

➤ The court must appoint a "guardian *ad litem*" or court evaluator, to bring the interests of the proposed ward to the attention of the court. In some states, the court appointee, often an attorney, serves as the proposed ward's personal advocate. In other states, the appointee functions as an independent investigator for the court.

➤ The person bringing the guardianship proceeding (the "petitioner") must comply with certain procedural requirements and notify the allegedly incapacitated person of the proceeding.

➤ The court, in its order of appointment, determines the scope of the guardian's authority. The authority can be broad and sweeping, or limited.

Take, for example, the case of Maggie, an eighty-five-year-old childless widow. When Maggie adamantly refused to enter a nursing home despite her niece's prodding, the niece commenced a guardianship proceeding. In her petition to the court, the niece requested permission to place her aunt in a nursing facility.

Maggie's niece explained to the court that Maggie could not remain in her own home. Electricity and telephone service had been cut off when Maggie didn't pay her bills, and the property had fallen into such disrepair that it was no longer habitable.

The court appointed the niece as the guardian of Maggie's property, to pay Maggie's bills and maintain her property, but it did not give the niece any control over Maggie's person. The niece could not control where her aunt lived or how she spent her days. The court limited the guardian's authority to financial management, since no evidence had been presented that Maggie could not care for her personal needs.

The court's decision to give the niece only that amount of authority necessary to protect Maggie's well-being reflects a judicial trend. Judges are exercising greater restraint in delegating authority to surrogate decision-makers, such as guardians. They are making a greater effort to match the delegation of authority with the incapacitated person's specific limitations.

In the health care context, guardianship proceedings are usually brought by a patient's family, friends, doctors, or medical facility. The goal of these proceedings is often to have a guardian appointed to direct the termination of life-sustaining medical treatment or resolve a dispute among feuding kin.

Guardianship proceedings are usually costly and time-consuming. On rare occasion, they can be avoided.

Take the case of Jamie Butcher, a thirty-four-year-old man who had been in a vegetative state since age seventeen. A Minnesota court allowed Jamie's parents to proceed with their plan to disconnect their son's feeding tube, even though they were never formally appointed their son's guardian.[126] The court used its equitable power to save the family the heart-wrenching ordeal of a full-blown guardianship proceeding.

FEDERAL RIGHT-TO-DIE LEGISLATION

Most issues of health care rights are covered by state law. Laws governing advance directives, guardianship proceedings, and surrogate decision making have been passed by state legislatures across the country. The federal government has not, however, remained completely silent. Federal right-to-die legislation, both implemented and proposed, is discussed below.

The U.S. Congress spoke up as an advocate for the widespread use of advance directives when it passed the Patient Self-Determination Act. The Patient Self-Determination Act (PSDA) of 1990 was enacted in direct response to the unfortunate plight of Nancy Cruzan's family (discussed on pages 149-150). In fact, the legislation was first introduced to Congress one day after the Missouri attorney general filed his U.S. Supreme Court brief in the *Cruzan* case. The legislation was an obvious response to nationwide concern about the efforts being made to artificially prolong life without regard to the patient's wishes and the compassionate practice of medicine.

The PSDA requires all health care facilities, including hospitals, hospices, home health agencies, and HMOs, that receive Medicare or Medicaid reimbursement to inform their patients, in writing, about the patient's right to refuse treatment and to prepare an advance medical directive. Providers are also required to educate their physicians, patients, staff, and the community about the availability and effect of advance directives. Finally, providers are required to inform incoming patients about any internal policies that limit the patient's right to refuse treatment (such as a facility's religious affiliation).

The law doesn't stop there. Health care providers who fall within the scope of the PSDA must also ask each and every patient whether he or she has signed an advance directive. If there is a directive, it must be incorporated into the patient's medical file and honored by the patient's doctors as required by state law. The providers may not, however, require the patient to sign an advance directive as a condition of admission to the facility or treatment.

Since most health care organizations receive some Medicare and/or Medicaid funds, the law is inclusive. Certified facilities that do not comply with the PSDA risk losing their Medicare and Medicaid reimbursement. The PSDA has both fans and detractors.

Supporters of the legislation credit the PSDA with encouraging families to discuss the dying process. By forcing patients to confront this difficult topic, they argue, the PSDA has returned health care decision making to the family. Families should be making treatment decisions instead of health care professionals who are more susceptible to the influences of their own economic considerations, patient biases, and religious values.

Critics of the PSDA point to poor enforcement as a significant weakness of the legislation. Nursing homes are the only class of medical facilities regularly monitored for compliance.

There is also some concern that the PSDA requires the wrong people to raise the wrong subjects at the wrong time. Should untrained personnel in the admissions office of the hospital really be asking incoming patients whether they want to be kept alive with tube feedings? Isn't a hospital or nursing home admission stressful enough, without bringing up the subject of death? Should personnel charged with discussing these topics be required to undergo sensitivity training?

It is important to recognize what the PSDA does *not* do: it does not expand patient rights. The law only educates patients and health care providers about the rights that already exist.

The American Bar Association (ABA) is urging the federal government to pass a substantive law to unify the rules governing health care decision-making for incapacitated patients. The patchwork of state laws and court decisions that determine who makes treatment decisions for patients who cannot make those decisions for themselves yields inconsistent outcomes and uncertainty. The ABA has drafted a proposed right-to-die law called the Uniform Health-Care Decisions Act, which it hopes will eventually replace conflicting state-specific rules and regulations.

The centerpiece of the Uniform Health-Care Decisions Act is a provision that authorizes every competent adult to prepare an advance directive. The law approves of both living wills and health care powers of attorney. Decision making for patients who lose capacity without having left specific directions regarding their care would be made by the patient's legal guardian.

RESOURCES

AARP Fulfillment (EE0888)
601 E Street, NW
Washington, D.C. 20049

The American Association of Retired Persons (AARP) publishes three booklets concerning medical decision making: Tomorrow's Choices *(stock #D13479),* Matter of Choice: Planning Ahead for Health Care Decision *(stock #D12776), and* Who Decides if You Can't *(stock #D15294). These books can be ordered at no charge from AARP.*

AARP's Legal Counsel for the Elderly (LCE) has also prepared two manuals. They are entitled Planning for Incapacity *(stock # is state-specific) and* Organizing Your Future: A Guide to Decision-Making in Your Later Years *(stock #D13877).* Planning for Incapacity *costs $5, and* Organizing Your Future *costs $12.95. Send check or money order to LCE/AARP, P.O. Box 96474, Washington, D.C. 20090-6474 (telephone number 202-434-2120). If ordering* Planning for Incapacity, *indicate your state of residence.*

Choice in Dying
200 Varick Street
New York, NY 10014-4810
1-800-989-WILL

Choice in Dying is a national not-for-profit organization that has as its mission protecting the rights of terminally ill patients and their families. Choice in Dying was formed when Concern for Dying merged with Society for the Right to Die.

Choice in Dying promotes the use of advance medical directives by providing at no charge state-specific directives to the public upon request. If you would like to receive a standard living will form or health care power of attorney or proxy that conforms to the law in your state, call or write Choice in Dying. In 1992, the organization sent out 400,000 form directives.

For a $25 annual membership fee you can join Choice in Dying. As a member *you will be notified of any changes in your state's law on medical directives, amended forms when needed, a card indicating that you have prepared an advance directive, and an annual subscription to* Choices, Choice in Dying's *quarterly newsletter.*

Choice in Dying also maintains a living will registry, which ensures that your living will will be available to your health care providers when needed. For a $40 registration fee, Choice in Dying will store a copy of your living will in a computer database and give you an identification card with the information necessary to access your document. Your health care provider will be able to call the registry's toll-free number and, using the information on your identification card, receive a copy of your living will by fax or computer transfer.

The following books pertain to medical decision making:

Final Passages: Positive Choices for the Dying and Their Loved Ones, by Judith Ahronheim (Simon and Schuster, 1992).

Deathright: Culture, Medicine, Politics, and the Right to Die, by James M. Hoefler (Westview Press, 1994).

Last Rights: Death Control and the Elderly in America, by Barbara J. Logue (Lexington Books, 1993).

SEVEN

Your Right to Assisted Suicide and Euthanasia

Do terminally ill, competent patients have the right to a doctor's assistance if they want to end their lives? Should doctors who prescribe a lethal dose of medication to patients suffering untreatable pain be protected from legal liability? What if the doctor administers the medication without the patient's explicit request? Should the doctor be charged with manslaughter, or praised as a humanitarian?

Most people already have strong feelings about these issues, but consider the following scenarios. They illustrate the complexity of these life-and-death questions.

Mary knows she is in the early stages of Alzheimer's disease. She has become increasingly forgetful and has even experienced fleeting periods of confusion. Mary is all too familiar with what lies ahead. She nursed her own mother for ten years while the disease ravaged the older woman's brain. Mary pledged never to let what happened to her mother happen to herself. She decided to ask her doctor for a lethal prescription of drugs that her son could help her take if she ever became completely disoriented. Should the doctor provide Mary with the prescription?

Mr. and Mrs. Kahn have been married for almost fifty years. As a result of a degenerative neurological condition, Mr. Kahn is in constant pain. The painkillers his doctors prescribed no longer relieve his suffering. Mr.

Kahn has told his wife on several occasions that if she loved him she would help him end his life. Mrs. Kahn finally starts to stockpile her husband's pain medications. She plans to cause her husband's death with an overdose of the drugs. Is Mrs. Kahn morally and ethically justified in helping her husband kill himself?

When John started to experience painful headaches at age thirty he joked about having a brain tumor. Tests eventually confirmed the presence of a large mass on his brain, and John's thoughts immediately turned to suicide. He could not tolerate the prospect of undergoing painful and debilitating radiation and chemotherapy treatments and becoming a burden to his family. He decided to ask his doctor for a lethal dose of medications. What should John's doctor do?

Phyllis lapsed into a coma following a massive stroke. She was completely nonresponsive. After a few months, her family asked the attending doctor to terminate the tube feedings and put an end to Phyllis's suffering. They told the doctor it was cruel to keep her body alive when there was no hope of recovery, and that Phyllis would not have wanted to be maintained on life support. When asked, the family admitted they had no proof of Phyllis's feelings about life support. The doctor refused to terminate the tube feedings. Did the doctor make the right decision?

Each of these four examples goes to the heart of the debate surrounding assisted suicide and euthanasia. The questions ask when, if at all, a doctor should help a patient commit suicide; they explore the difficulties of proving a patient's competency to decide to end his or her life; and they highlight the special problems posed by incompetent patients who cannot make choices about their own declining health.

In order to formulate reasoned answers to all of these questions, you must be able to distinguish between assisted suicide, euthanasia, and the right to refuse medical treatment. While all three terms relate to death and dying, they are far from synonymous.

Assisted suicide occurs when someone helps another individual bring about his or her own death. A doctor who gives a patient a prescription for a lethal dose of medication, for example, participates in assisted suicide. The doctor helps the patient take his or her own life by means of a drug overdose.

Euthanasia, or mercy killing, has nothing to do with suicide. Euthanasia occurs when one person causes another person's death without that person's participation. A doctor who decides to inject a fatal dose of morphine into an incompetent patient's arm performs euthanasia.

The right to refuse treatment is distinct from assisting suicide or causing another's death. The right to refuse treatment refers to each individual's constitutionally protected right to determine what shall, and shall not, be done to his or her body. While we are competent, no one can interfere with our decision to accept or refuse a recommended medical treatment. If we become incapacitated, our prior expressions of health care preferences continue to control the care we receive. The right to refuse treatment is explored in depth in chapter 6 and will not be covered in this chapter.

What makes the issue of assisted suicide such a hot topic of public discourse are the strong competing interests at stake. The medical profession, society, and patients themselves all have reason to care deeply about the outcome of the debate.

Doctors have an interest in preserving life. From the day incoming medical students register for anatomy class through their internship, residency, and fellowship, they are taught to heal the sick. Death becomes the enemy, and the loss of a patient is often taken as a personal defeat.

Given this indoctrination, it should be expected that many doctors are repulsed by the prospect of participating in a patient's death. After all, new doctors pledge to "first, do not harm" when they take the Hippocratic oath.

It should come as no surprise, for example, that the American Medical Association (AMA) elevates the interest of the medical profession in treating sickness over the interests of the state and individual. The official position of the AMA's Council on Ethical and Judicial Affairs is that "[p]hysicians must not perform euthanasia or participate in assisted suicide."[127] Doctors do their job when they use their medical know-how to relieve the pain and suffering that leads many patients to consider suicide. The job of doctors is not to hasten death.

Doctors practicing medicine in the trenches are far from unanimous in their support of the AMA's stance on assisted suicide. In fact, a study published in *The New England Journal of Medicine* showed the medical profession to be sharply divided over the issue.

Half of the doctors surveyed said physicians were sometimes justified in helping a patient die by administering a drug overdose, while 39 percent said such action was never ethically justified. Though 53 percent of doctors thought physician-assisted suicide should be legal, only 40 percent said they would be willing to help a patient die.

The study showed support for assisted suicide to be split along the lines of medical specialty, gender, and religious affiliation. Blood and cancer specialists, the doctors most likely to have contact with terminally ill patients, were the strongest opponents of assisted suicide. Psychiatrists, who had the least exposure to terminally ill patients, were the strongest advocates of the practice. Female physicians were significantly more likely to support assisted suicide than male doctors were. Fifty-six percent of those who opposed assisted suicide said their opinions were influenced by religious beliefs.

In an effort to make the practice of physician-assisted suicide more palatable to the medical profession, a group of eight Michigan doctors calling themselves Physicians for Mercy have proposed ten regulatory guidelines for the practice. Under the guidelines, doctors could only assist in a suicide if certain specialists agreed that the patient was mentally competent, afflicted with an incurable condition, suffering uncontrollable agony, and could not tolerate the side effects of pain management and medical therapy. Initial reaction to the guidelines, according to spokespeople for the medical profession, ranged from negative to skeptical.

States, like doctors, also have a vested interest in the legality of assisted suicide. States are responsible for protecting the well-being of their residents. When a resident is incapable of caring for herself, and is at risk of harm, the state is obligated to step in and provide that resident with the care she needs. Similarly, when a resident is suffering physical or emotional pain, and may be inclined to take her own life, the state has the duty to discourage that resident from committing suicide. Criminalizing assisted suicide is one way many states protect the lives of their residents.

Last, but certainly not least, are the interests of patients in legalizing assisted suicide. The suicide rate among Americans age 65 and older increased 9 percent from 1980 to 1982, according to the Federal Centers for Disease Control and Prevention. The interests of doctors in fighting death, and the interests of society in protecting life, are rivaled by the interests of patients in controlling their personal destiny.

When June, at age seventy-six, was told by her doctor that the cancer previously confined to her thyroid had spread throughout her body, she knew what she had to do. Both her mother and husband had died from cancer. June refused to suffer the same fate. She elected not to undergo disfiguring surgery that gave her only a slim chance of survival, and she decided instead to contact Compassion in Dying, a Seattle-based group that counsels people who want help ending their lives.[128] If June had to die, she wanted to orchestrate the circumstances of her death.

There is evidence that the public believes that patients should have the right to ask for help in ending their lives when they have decided enough is enough. A 1995 poll of Michigan residents, for example, found that 66 percent of respondents supported the legalization of assisted suicide. Membership in the Hemlock Society, a group that promotes euthanasia or "mercy killing," has skyrocketed in recent years. A book entitled *Final Exit: The Practicalities of Self-Deliverance and Assisted Suicide for the Dying* quickly made it onto the best-seller lists.[129] Despite this yearning for control, many people fear that the availability of physician-assisted suicide will weaken the human spirit.

John, a thirty-five-year-old executive, is diagnosed with acute myelocytic leukemia. His doctor tells him that he has a 25 percent chance of survival with medical treatment. Without treatment, he will die within months. He starts thinking about taking his own life. A quick and painless death seems preferable to becoming dependent on his wife, turning into a monster in the eyes of his young children as his appearance changes, depleting the nest egg his family worked so hard to save, and suffering through chemotherapy and radiation.

In this example, John is more troubled by the *process* of dying than death itself.

John's reaction to his diagnosis is not unusual. For many terminally ill patients, fears of embarrassment, pain, and loss of independence and control are prominent.

Without the option of physician-assisted suicide, dying patients have no choice. They must endure the dying process. As part of this process, they often lean on friends and family for support. Some ponder their accomplishments and regrets. Conversation and personal reflection enable many terminally ill patients to accept death, rather than fear it to the bitter end.

Patients may avoid this difficult process if suicide is presented to them as an option. They may opt for a quick and painless physician-assisted suicide, and die without enduring the emotional and spiritual trial of the dying process.

Another risk associated with legalizing assisted suicide is the so-called slippery slope. Once doctors are permitted to bring to a premature end the lives of their terminally ill mentally competent patients, will they soon be allowed to hasten the death of terminally ill patients who do not request any assistance in ending their lives? Will they then be allowed to kill off chronically ill patients, physically disabled patients, psychologically distressed patients, and ultimately any undesirable patient?

The slippery slope argument is premised on what is probably an incorrect assumption: that doctors do not know the moral difference between helping people bring their suffering to an end and killing people who want to live. Advocates of physician-assisted suicide counter that doctors are at greater risk of losing their moral footing if they continue to be legally required to ignore the pleas of patients who beg for a humane end to their pain and suffering.

Many people are quick to associate assisted suicide with Dr. Jack Kevorkian. Dr. Kevorkian is a retired pathologist who has helped at least twenty-seven people take their own lives. He helped these individuals commit suicide without ever having treated them as patients, and without regard to their anticipated life expectancy.

There is a danger in drawing any conclusions about assisted suicide based on the activities of Dr. Kevorkian. Every suicide assist is not created equal. Consider, for example, another doctor's resort to assisted suicide.

Dr. Timothy Quill, a Rochester internist, decided to help a terminally ill patient commit suicide after years of treating her for leukemia. The doctor publicized his decision to prescribe a lethal dose of sleeping pills to "Diane" in *The New England Journal of Medicine*.[130] In the journal article, the doctor described the severity of Diane's illness, his inability to mitigate her pain with medication, and the painstaking process by which he became convinced that Diane was competent to make a rational decision to end her life.

This chapter will explore the nuances of assisted suicide and euthanasia. The goal of the chapter is to examine the rights of patients to bring an end to their suffering, and to consider the legal and political challenges our judges and legislators face in defining those rights.

JUDICIALLY DEFINED RIGHTS

Here's an interesting question. People have been dying for as long as there have been people. Why are decade-old laws prohibiting assisted suicide only coming under attack now? Why have we waited so long to demand our doctors' help in ending our lives?

The answer probably lies in the medical profession's unprecedented ability to prolong life. Fantastic advances in medical technology enable doctors to hold death at bay, leaving patients to question whether the additional days, months, or years of life are worth the attendant pain, expense, and lost quality of life.

The deterioration of the doctor-patient relationship has not helped matters. Patients are more wary than ever of their doctors' intentions. Patients and doctors no longer enjoy the bonds of loyalty and respect that characterized their relationship in the past. With the diminishing presence of the family physician and the increasing use of specialists, patients have achieved an unprecedented alienation from their doctors. Add to this a sense among patients that corporate executives, insurance company administrators, and malpractice attorneys are influencing the decisions that doctors are making, and you have a breeding ground for mistrust and skepticism.

The significance of the legal debate surrounding the right to assisted suicide can not be overstated. By the time all is said and done, the U.S. Supreme Court might establish a new constitutional right to assisted suicide. This right could be premised on rights recognized decades earlier in connection with a woman's right to terminate a pregnancy.

The link between the divisive issues of abortion and assisted suicide may not be immediately apparent. Sure, both issues concern life and death, but one has to do with the beginning of life and the other has to do with the end of life. What's the connection?

The connection, in the opinion of one judge, is that the right to terminate a pregnancy and the right to bring one's own life to an end are both "[m]atters involving the most intimate and personal choices a person may make in a lifetime." In 1994, Washington's U. S. District Court judge Barbara Rothstein drew the parallel between abortion and assisted suicide in a case called *Compassion in Dying*,[131] which challenged the constitutionality of that state's ban on assisted suicide.[132]

In *Compassion in Dying v. Washington*, Judge Rothstein took a historical look at abortion rights cases. She concluded that the same reasoning that supports a woman's right to a doctor's assistance in aborting an unwanted fetus supports a terminally ill patient's right to a doctor's assistance in hastening death. She further found that just as states are free to regulate a woman's right to terminate a pregnancy, states are free to regulate physician-assisted suicide.

Compassion in Dying has come to be known as the *Roe v. Wade* of the right-to-die movement. It is the first declaration of a new constitutional right to assisted suicide.

In March 1995, Judge Rothstein's ruling was reversed on appeal. Washington's ban on assisted suicide was upheld as constitutional.[133] The appellate court held that doctor-assisted suicide was "antithetical to the defense of human life that has been a chief responsibility of our constitutional government."[134]

One year later, in March 1996, a higher federal appeals court agreed with Judge Rothstein. The Ninth U.S. Circuit Court of Appeals ruled that Washington State's ban on doctor-assisted suicide was unconstitutional. According to the appellate panel, the state's duty to preserve life is outweighed by the right to control "the time and manner of one's death." The State Attorney General has the right to appeal this decision to the U.S. Supreme Court.

If the Supreme Court eventually accepts Judge Rothstein's reasoning, the right of patients to physician-assisted suicide will be analogous to the present right of pregnant women to abort a fetus. The right will not be absolute. Just as a woman's right to have an abortion depends on the law in her state and the stage of gestation, so a patient's right to physician-assisted suicide will depend on the relevant state law and the precise nature of the patient's physical and mental condition.

Decade-old arguments made in connection with abortion are also now starting to be made in connection with euthanasia. Matthew Habiger, president of Human Life International, an anti-abortion advocacy organization, explicitly connected the two issues: "The march toward a complete anti-life philosophy can now be easily mapped: from contraception to abortion to euthanasia."

A newfound constitutional right to physician-assisted suicide would surely come with associated risks. The primary risk would be that states would fail to adequately regulate suicide assists. Inadequate regulation would allow doctors to accede to the wishes of clinically depressed patients who requested an expedient end to their suffering. Elderly, poor, and minority patients would be especially vulnerable to pressure to bring their lives to a quick end.

In reality, the Supreme Court is unlikely to find a constitutional right to assisted suicide. The High Court is more likely to follow the leads of the New York and Michigan courts, both of which upheld the constitutionality of criminal bans against assisting suicide. In Michigan, the court explicitly found that the constitutional rights established in earlier decisions concerning abortion were inapplicable to assisted suicide.[135] The New York judge, in his decision upholding that state's ban on assisted suicide (a decision now on appeal), relied on the state's "obvious legitimate interest in preserving life and in protecting vulnerable persons."[136]

Although patients living in states that have a statutory ban on physician-assisted suicide do not have any right to ask their doctor for help committing suicide, they may have the right to ask their doctor to take measures to relieve their suffering, even if those measures hasten their death. Consider the case of Thomas W. Hyde, Jr., a thirty-year-old man suffering from amyotrophic lateral sclerosis, who went to Dr. Kevorkian seeking relief from his pain.

These are the undisputed facts of the case: On August 4, 1993, Dr. Kevorkian placed a mask over Mr. Hyde's face. The doctor then gave Mr. Hyde, who was nearly paralyzed, a string to pull to release a flow of carbon monoxide gas. Mr. Hyde died as a direct result of his inhalation of the toxic fumes. One month before his death, Mr. Hyde had videotaped himself expressing a wish to die.

The prosecution's argument to the jury was simple. If they believed that Mr. Hyde committed suicide, and that Dr. Kevorkian provided him with the means to commit suicide, they would have to find Dr. Kevorkian guilty of violating Michigan's now expired law against assisting in a suicide. Any sympathy the jury might have for Mr. Hyde could not play a role in their decision.

Dr. Kevorkian's attorney argued that his client was innocent. He based his argument on a clause in the state's assisted suicide ban that allowed a doctor to take measures to relieve a patient's suffering, even if those measures hastened the patient's death. Mr. Fieger asked the jury to find that Dr. Kevorkian's intention in fitting Mr. Hyde with the carbon monoxide mask was to relieve suffering, not cause death. If the jury reached this conclusion, Fieger argued, Dr. Kevorkian could not be found guilty of illegally assisting suicide.

On May 2, 1994 (one day before Washington judge Rothstein rendered her decision in *Compassion in Dying*), after about ten hours of deliberations, the jury came back with a verdict: Not guilty. The jury had accepted the defense attorney's argument that Dr. Kevorkian had not broken a now expired Michigan law[137] that prohibited the act of helping another person die, since the doctor's primary goal had been to relieve Mr. Hyde's suffering, not cause his death.[138]

The jury's decision in the Kevorkian case was widely interpreted as a de facto referendum on assisted suicide. In acquitting Kevorkian, the jurors effectively communicated their support of allowing seriously ill patients who are competent to decide their fate to obtain assistance in ending their lives. On March 8, 1996, a second jury acquitted Dr. Kevorkian under the same law.

At the very least, Dr. Kevorkian's acquittals highlight the difficulty of distinguishing legitimate medical procedures that unintentionally cause or hasten the patient's death from those acts that are intended to result in the patient's death. The distinction assumes tremendous significance under both the law and medical ethics.

Doctors are permitted to prescribe pain-relieving medications that may increase a patient's risk of death, just as they are allowed to recommend high-risk surgical procedures. As long as the recommendation is made with the intent of improving the patient's quality of life and not causing the patient's death, the doctor acts within the relevant moral and legal boundaries. The only requirement is that the doctor advise the patient of any known risks before commencing the treatment.

The jury's characterization of Dr. Kevorkian's administration of a lethal dose of carbon monoxide as a legitimate medical treatment is, at best, a stretch. The prosecution was probably correct in concluding that the emotion of the case clouded the jury's ability to apply the law. The jurors may well have been sending a message to Dr. Kevorkian: Stay out of jail so you can help us commit suicide if we are ever facing a life of relentless pain.

The line between a legitimate medical treatment and a suicide assist might not have been so blurry in the jury's mind if Kevorkian had not been a physician— albeit a pathologist not trained in patient care who also happened to have lost his medical licence a few years earlier. If someone other than a doctor had helped Mr. Hyde take his own life, the act might have been more clearly perceived to be a suicide assist.

That the distinction between palliative care and assisted suicide is unclear is beyond dispute. Take, for example, the morphine drip. The morphine drip is a slow, continuous injection of a painkiller into a vein.

Doctors start morphine drips to relieve the pain of their patients. Morphine drips can, however, cause death by curtailing respiration when administered at high doses and for extended periods of time. A patient's death from a morphine drip is an unintended, but foreseeable, consequence of the use of the drip.

Many doctors who do not overtly participate in assisted suicide or euthanasia readily resort to the morphine drip when a patient is dying. Even the Catholic Church approves of the practice. According to a 1975 directive from the National Conference of Catholic Bishops, "It is not euthanasia to give a dying person sedatives and analgesics for the alleviation of pain even though they may deprive the patient of the use of reason, or shorten his life." Tens of thousands of morphine drips are started each year across the country.

In the opinion of some medical ethicists, a morphine drip is undeniably euthanasia. The confusion stems from the fact that the morphine drip does not conform to the popular understanding of euthanasia.

When most people think of euthanasia they think of an act that brings about the patient's immediate death. Few would dispute, for example, that a physician who injects a patient with a large dose of morphine is practicing euthanasia. With a morphine drip, the patient's death is gradual. While the patient is dying, everything else proceeds as normal. Loved ones continue to visit. Hospital staff check in on the patient. Since the doctor is rarely present, the connection between the physician and the direct cause of death is severed.

Starting a morphine drip is also not characterized as an act of euthanasia because the stated purpose of the drip is to ease a patient's suffering. Using a morphine drip to control pain is accepted medical practice. Only when the morphine drip is used to end a patient's life is the treatment illegal and unethical. In the opinion of some medical ethicists, this distinction is a myth. Doctors know that the morphine drip will hasten the patient's death, whether or not that is the stated purpose of the treatment.

The medical profession's failure to honestly confront the true nature of the morphine drip arguably breeds deception, medical paternalism, and inequality of treatment. There is deception when a doctor commences a "treatment" that he knows, but does not say, is sure to end in the patient's death. There is medical paternalism when a doctor, rather than the patient or the patient's family, decides it is time to "start the drip" and hasten the patient's death. Finally, there is a risk of inequitable care when doctors have sole authority to make the highly discretionary determination about using a morphine drip.

Although some state statutes prohibit assisted suicide while permitting the administration of life-shortening palliative care, such as the morphine drip, other states have no assisted suicide statute at all. Even where the state legislature has failed to prohibit assisted suicide, the legality of the act is questionable. For proof, take a quick look at another of Dr. Kevorkian's legal entanglements.

Some of Dr. Kevorkian's suicide assists occurred at a time when Michigan did not have a state ban against the practice. Michigan prosecutors, desperate for a legal hook with which to charge Dr. Kevorkian with a crime, looked to a 1920 murder case. The case involved a husband who placed poison within his ill wife's reach when his wife asked for his help in ending her life. The defendant husband was successfully prosecuted for his wife's murder.

When Dr. Kevorkian's lawyer learned that criminal charges had been filed against his client based on the common-law crime of murder, he characterized the decision as "amazingly goofy" (a phrase not likely to be found in Black's Law Dictionary). In December 1994 the Michigan Supreme Court ruled that assisting in suicide was a crime of murder based on the common law. Although the U.S. Supreme Court refused to hear Dr. Kevorkian's appeal, in August 1995 a Michigan judge dismissed the murder charges, finding that the prosecution had failed to prove all of the necessary elements of a murder charge.

LEGISLATIVELY DEFINED RIGHTS

On the morning of July 31, 1991, sixty-five-year-old William F. Meyer III summoned police to the home of his eighty-eight-year-old father, William F. Meyer Jr. When the police arrived they found that Mr. Meyer Jr. was dead. A plastic bag was wrapped around his head, and a suicide note was found near his body. The note read, "I happily decided that it was more kind and thoughtful of me to terminate my life before I reached a decadent condition of helplessness." The police offered their sympathies to the younger Mr. Meyer, and concluded that the older man had decided to end his own life.

Two months later the police were back to arrest Mr. Meyer III. They had read a published interview with Mr. Meyer III wherein the son described how he had planned to tie a bag around his father's head and how his father's longtime physician had agreed to prescribe enough painkillers to ensure that Mr. Meyer Jr. would be asleep by the time the oxygen in the bag ran out. The younger Mr. Meyer, a sales executive and leader of his church, was charged with second-degree manslaughter. If convicted, he faced ten years in prison.[139]

This true story illustrates the important distinction between the legality of ending, or attempting to end, one's own life and the legality of helping another individual end his or her life. Whereas no state in the nation criminalizes the act of suicide, most jurisdictions do criminalize the act of assisting another's suicide.

A push to remove this legislative distinction is underway.

Poll after poll shows people wanting greater control over the circumstances of their death. They want to reclaim from their doctors the right to decide when they have suffered enough pain, and when it is time to bring their lives of suffering to a humane and dignified end.

Support for legalizing assisted suicide is apparent upon review of the public's response to legislative initiatives to legalize assisted suicide. In 1991 and 1993 attempts to pass legislation legalizing physician-assisted suicide were narrowly defeated in the states of Washington and California. On November 8, 1994, Oregon voters approved the nation's first law sanctioning physician-assisted suicide.

Prior to the passage of Oregon's so-called Measure 16, assisted suicide had been a felony in Oregon, as in most other states in the country. The Oregon law, which was scheduled to take effect on December 8, 1994, protects from legal liability those doctors who in "good faith" follow its guidelines in prescribing lethal doses of drugs to terminally ill patients who request them. The law leaves to each individual doctor the decision about whether or not to comply with a patient's request to die.

The Oregon statute includes several restrictions that are intended to guard against abuse. A doctor is only permitted to hasten the death of a terminally ill patient who has six months or less to live in the opinion of at least two physicians. The patient's doctor and one other physician must also agree that the patient is mentally competent to decide to commit suicide. The patient must ask for help ending his or her life on at least three separate occasions, with the last request made in writing. After the final request is made, the doctor is required to wait fifteen days before providing the patient with the lethal prescription. Only Oregon residents who are at least eighteen years of age and have lived in the state for at least one year are covered by the law.

The bill to legalize assisted suicide that passed in Oregon, unlike the measures that were defeated in Washington and California, involves the physician only to the extent that the physician prescribes the fatal drug. The patient must self-administer the medication in the presence of two eyewitnesses. Legislation proposed in the other states allowed doctors to help administer the lethal dose of the drugs. Perhaps this difference explains the favorable response of the Oregon voters.

The reaction to the passage of Measure 16 in Oregon, has been mixed, to say the least. So-called right-to-die groups have celebrated in triumph. "Right-to-life" groups and the Roman Catholic Church have condemned the Oregon vote as "a day of mourning for all humanity." Catholic hospitals in Oregon promptly announced that they would not be allowing assisted suicide in their facilities. In making strange bedfellows with the Catholic Church, Dr. Kevorkian also came out against the Oregon effort. He criticized the law for only giving terminally ill patients the right to get help ending their lives; quality of life, not life expectancy, should control the availability of suicide assistance, according to Kevorkian.

Many people have openly displayed shock and horror at the idea of state-sanctioned suicide. They believe that giving people an easy way out of their suffering weakens the human spirit. They fear that the valued tradition of supporting and comforting loved ones as they gradually approach the end of life will be lost as more and more seriously ill patients opt for an expeditious suicide. They worry that the sick will cut their lives short out of concern that they have become a burden or an embarrassment to others.

Some opponents of assisted suicide blame baby boomers for passage of the Oregon law. Baby boomers, as a group, are reputed to lust after power and instant gratification. Legalized assisted suicide promises patients more control and faster results in connection with their impending deaths. These promises, the argument goes, may be intuitively attractive to many young baby boomers who have had little real life experience with death and dying.

Perhaps the greatest fear associated with the legalization of physician-assisted suicide is that the law will be inequitably applied. There is overwhelming evidence that all Americans do not enjoy equal access to the nation's health care resources. Study after study shows that minorities receive inferior medical care in this country. Many citizens who lack adequate health care coverage cannot afford to see a doctor when they are sick, or enter a clean and well-staffed hospital when they require inpatient treatment. In this climate of inequality, legalizing doctor-assisted suicide is seen as an invitation to disaster. Will undesirable patients be pressured to take their own lives?

The Oregon law illustrates the inherent problem of defining a statutory right to physician-assisted suicide.

Which patients should fall within the scope of the law allowing physician-assisted suicide? Oregon legislators decided that only patients whose death was expected within six months could ask for a doctor's help in committing suicide. But is six months too long? Predicting life expectancy is not a perfect science. Physicians may be able to accurately predict how long someone will live when it's a matter of days or even weeks, but patients who are given six months to live often live much longer. Also, six months is long enough for doctors to find a new treatment, improve pallative measures, or for the patient to find new meaning in life.

What procedural safeguards are needed to ensure that doctors do not abuse their power and wrongfully hasten the death of their patients? The Oregon law only requires the consent of a second physician. Should the consent of an independently referred doctor be required before the patient's request for assistance is granted? Should the decision then be reviewed by a panel of medical ethicists? Are doctors too likely to rubber-stamp the decisions of their colleagues?

On December 7, 1994, one day before the Oregon law allowing doctor-assisted suicide was to take effect, a Federal District Court judge blocked implementation.

At the time of publication, a decision had not yet been rendered on the legality of the Oregon initiative. A number of constitutional issues remain to be resolved.

Before the Oregon legislation legalizing assisted suicide was blocked, speculation ran rampant as to how many people would request their doctor's help in committing suicide once the practice was decriminalized. Would Oregonian doctors be overwhelmed with requests? Would Oregon, the Beaver State, become known as the Death State? One study based on interviews with terminally ill patients and another country's experience with legalized assisted suicide concluded that no more than 2 percent of patients facing imminent death were likely to request assistance in committing suicide.

If you were seriously ill and in intense pain, would you take advantage of a law that gave you a statuatory right to your doctor's assistance in ending your life? Or would you prefer to have your doctor administer comfort care once there was no likelihood you could be cured?

Medical schools have traditionally emphasized treatment and deemphasized effective pain management. The legislative push to legalize physician-assisted suicide may well lose steam if doctors are taught to administer higher and more frequent doses of painkilling medications, even if the effect of the drugs is to hasten death.

When a patient is going to die regardless of what the doctor does, many doctors reluctantly concede defeat. They eventually accept that medicine has failed this patient, and turn away from the dying patient to focus their energies on saving patients who still stand a chance of winning the battle against death.

This problem of abandonment will change only if medical schools start teaching new doctors how to ease the physical and emotional suffering of their dying patients. Until doctors are better trained to treat the pain and depression that lead most patients to seek an expeditious death, the push to legalize assisted suicide and euthanasia is unlikely to abate.

The conflict between physician-assisted suicide and the medical treatment of pain came head-to-head in November 1994 when Dr. Kevorkian responded to charges that he had refused to allow two mainstream doctors to treat the pain of a woman whom Kevorkian later helped commit suicide. The woman, Margaret Garrish, a seventy-two-year-old homemaker, was suffering from rheumatoid arthritis, advanced osteoporosis, severe colon disorders, and other ailments when she asked Dr. Kevorkian to help her commit suicide. The doctors who offered to treat Ms. Garrish's pain pointed out that Dr. Kevorkian could not prescribe painkilling drugs himself, since his license to practice medicine was suspended in 1991 after he began assisting in suicides.

Dr. Kevorkian said that the two doctors who had offered their assistance were opportunists. Publicity seekers. He noted that Ms. Garrish was already being treated with morphine patches for her pain, and that patches were losing their effect. One of the doctors, an anesthesiologist who specializes in pain management, responded that "there's a lot more we can do these days than morphine patches." The anesthesiologist related an anecdote about a former cancer patient who initially wanted Dr. Kevorkian's assistance in committing suicide but changed his mind after the anesthesiologist succeeded in relieving the patient's pain.

The idea that doctors should make dying patients comfortable, as opposed to treating their underlying medical condition or abandoning them entirely, is the underpinning of the hospice movement. Hospice workers are generally opposed to assisted suicide. The Oregon Hospice Association came out against the ballot initiative to legalize assisted suicide in that state. Legalizing assisted suicide, many hospice workers believe, will divert attention away from the medical profession's responsibility of easing the dying process. If the accepted mode of treating a terminally ill patient becomes bringing that patient's life to a quick end, fewer doctors will help their patients through the pain and psychological trauma of the death.

Many hospice advocates do, however, see a benefit in the attention that has been focused on assisted suicide. They see a clear message being sent to the medical profession that people want more control over their pain. According to Ann Jackson, director of the Oregon Hospice Association, the approval of Measure 16 by the Oregon voters was "a wake up call to the health care profession, and they had better listen."

After studying assisted suicide for two years, the New York State Task Force on Life and the Law advocated aggressive pain treatment. The task force was convened by former Governor Cuomo to consider whether physician-assisted suicide should be legalized in New York State. In concluding that it should not, the task force recommended that doctors provide their dying patients with medication to ease pain and depression, even if the medications hasten death.

In addition, the task force recommended that legislative action be taken to remove the stigma of using painkillers. New York law currently requires health workers to report addicts to the Health Department. As long as this legislation remains intact, doctors will not be free to respond to their patients' request for pain medication.

The task force also recommended that health care providers be taught the difference between the legal act of providing patients with palliative treatments that may lead to death and the illegal acts of assisting suicide and euthanasia. A doctor who gives painkilling medication that incidentally hastens death does not commit a crime under New York law. Without this education, doctors will remain fearful of prescribing more frequent or stronger pain medication. They will continue to wonder and worry. What if the additional medication slows the patient's respiration? What if the patient dies from respiratory distress? Will I go to jail?

The task force expressed a strong preference for improving the care provided to dying patients over legalizing physician-assisted suicide. According to Dr. Mark Chassin, the New York State health commissioner and task force member, "When you consider doctors' poor records at diagnosing and treating depression and our failure to adequately treat pain, you have to worry that patients would be inappropriately granted assisted suicide instead of having their depression and pain treated without being killed."

While unanimously opposing the idea of legalizing assisted suicide, the task force accepted that assisting suicide was moral and ethical under certain circumstances. The task force concluded, however, that the exceptional needs of the relatively small number of competent terminally ill patients who suffer untreatable pain should not determine public policy.

In its report, the task force painted a picture of a regulatory nightmare if New York legalized assisted suicide only in cases where the patient was near death, in severe pain, and free of suicidal depression. Of particular concern was how to set standards to uniformly predict life expectancy, how to independently verify the extent of someone else's subjective pain, and how to conclusively ascertain whether a patient who asks to die is suffering from depression.

The task force, while concluding that physician-assisted suicide should not be legally sanctioned, left the door open for terminally ill patients in severe pain to ask their doctors for help in hastening death. In a public dialogue with Dr. Quill, the Rochester physician who helped one of his longtime patients commit suicide, a task force member expressed hope that physicians would decide in private whether or not to accede to the wishes of competent terminally ill patients with uncontrollable pain who asked for help in ending their lives.

Patients should keep this important qualification in mind. Just because state legislators decide that legalizing physician-assisted suicide is bad public policy does not mean that the practice is not moral and appropriate under certain limited circumstances. The decision is ultimately one that must be made between an individual patient and his or her doctor. Remember that Dr. Quill, who publicized his decision to help a patient take her life, was neither disciplined by the State Board for Professional Medical Conduct nor indicted by a grand jury on criminal charges.

What are your feelings about physician-assisted suicide? When a doctor helps a patient end his life, is that doctor abandoning the patient or helping the patient? Will patients who want pain relief and comfort while they are dying be encouraged to commit suicide if assisted suicide is legalized? Are there patients for whom dying is the best course of care? Can assisted suicide be adequately regulated to guard against abuse?

Perhaps the best solution, as is often the case, is a compromise. Maybe physician-assisted suicide should be one of the palliatives that are available to dying people. If so, care must be taken to ensure that it does not become the hair-trigger response to the plight of dying people. The practice of assisted suicide can be tolerated only when it follows a careful analysis of the specific facts of an individual case. Assisted suicide cannot be judged to be an acceptable medical practice based on abstractions and general legal principals.

RESOURCES

If you are interested in obtaining additional information about assisted suicide or euthanasia, you can contact the following advocacy organizations:

PRO-ASSISTED SUICIDE/EUTHANASIA

Compassion in Dying
P.O. Box 75295
Seattle, WA 98125-0295
206-624-2775

Elisabeth Kübler-Ross Center
South Route 616
Head Waters, VA 24442
703-396-3441

National Hemlock Society
P.O. Box 11830
Eugene, OR 97440-3900
503-342-5748

ANTI-ASSISTED SUICIDE/EUTHANASIA

Americans United for Life
343 S. Dearborn, Suite 1804
Chicago, IL 60604
312-786-9494

International Anti-Euthanasia Task Force
Family Living Council
P.O. Box 760
Steubenville, OH 43952
614-282-3810

Secretariat for Pro-Life Activities
National Conference of Catholic Bishops
3211 4th Street, NE
Washington, D.C. 20017-1194
202-541-3070

The books listed below deal with the issues of death and dying:

Deadly Compassion, by Rita Marker (William Morrow, 1993).

How We Die: Reflections on Life's Final Chapter, by Sherwin Nuland (Knopf, 1994).

Life Work, by Donald Hall (Beacon Press, 1993).

Intoxicated by My Illness, by Anatole Broyard (Fawcett, 1992).

Coping with the Final Tragedy: Cultural variation in dying and grieving, edited by David and Dorothy Counts (Baywood, 1991).

The Death of Ivan Ilyich, by Leo Tolstoy (Penguin Classics, 1989).

On Death and Dying, by Elisabeth Kübler-Ross (Macmillan, 1970).

The American Way of Death, by Jessica Mitford (Simon and Schuster, 1963).

A Death in the Family, by James Agee (McDowell, Obolensky, 1957).

Death Be Not Proud, by John Gunther (Harper and Brothers, 1949).

APPENDICES

APPENDIX 1

State-by-State Listing of Departments of Health

Alabama

Department of Public Health
434 Monroe Street
Montgomery, AL 36130

Alaska

Department of Health and Social
  Services
P.O. Box 110610
Juneau, AK 99811

Arizona

Department of Health Services
1740 W. Adams Street
Phoenix, AZ 85007

Arkansas

Department of Health
4815 W. Markham Street
Little Rock, AR 72205

California

Department of Health Services
714 P Street
Sacramento, CA 95814

Colorado

Department of Health
4300 Cherry Creek Drive South
Denver, CO 80222

Connecticut

Department of Health Services
150 Washington Street
Hartford, CT 06106

Delaware

Department of Health and Social
  Services
P.O. Box 637
Dover, DE 19903

District of Columbia

Department of Human Services
1660 L Street, N.W.
Washington, D.C. 20036

Florida

Department of Health and
  Rehabilitative Services
1317 Winewood Boulevard
Tallahassee, FL 32399

Georgia

Department of Human Resources,
  Public Health Division
2 Peachtree Street
Atlanta, GA 30303

Hawaii

Department of Health
P.O. Box 3378
Honolulu, HI 96801

Idaho

Department of Health and Welfare
450 W. State Towers
Boise, ID 83720

Illinois

Department of Public Health
535 W. Jefferson Street
Springfield, IL 62761

Indiana

State Board of Health
1330 W. Michigan Street
Indianapolis, IN 46206

Iowa

Department of Public Health
Lucas State Office Building
Des Moines, IA 50319

Kansas

Department of Health and
Environment
900 S. W. Jackson
Topeka, KS 66612

Kentucky

Department of Health Services
275 E. Main Street
Frankfort, KY 40601

Louisiana

Department of Health and Hospitals
P.O. Box 3214
New Orleans, LA 70821

Maine

Department of Human Services
State House Station #11
Augusta, ME 04333

Maryland

Department of Health and Mental
Hygiene
201 W. Presont Street
Baltimore, MD 21201

Massachusetts

Department of Public Health
150 Tremon Street
Boston, MA 02111

Michigan

Department of Public Health
3500 N. Logan
P.O. Box 30035
Lansing, MI 48909

Minnesota

Department of Health
717 Delaware Street, S.E.
P.O. Box 9441
Minneapolis, MN 55440

Mississippi

Department of Health
2423 N. State Street
Jackson, MS 39216

Missouri

Department of Health
P.O. Box 570
Jefferson City, MO 65102

Montana

Department of Health and
Environmental Sciences
Cogswell Building
Helena, MT 59620

Nebraska

Department of Health
P.O. Box 95007
Lincoln, NE 68509

Nevada

Department of Human Resources,
   Health Division
505 E. King Street
Carson, City, NV 89710

New Hampshire

Department of Health and Human
   Services
Annex Building 1
115 Pleasant Street
Concord, NH 03301

New Jersey

Department of Health
John Fitch Plaza, CN 360
Trenton, NJ 08625

New Mexico

Department of Health
1190 St. Francis Drive
Santa Fe, MN 87502

New York

Department of Health
Corning Tower
Empire State Plaza
Albany, NY 12237

North Carolina

Department of Environment, Health
   and Natural Resources
P.O. Box 27687
Raleigh, NC 27611

North Dakota

Department of Health
600 E. Boulevard Avenue
Bismarck, ND 58505

Ohio

Department of Health
246 N. High Street
P.O. Box 118
Columbus, OH 43266

Oklahoma

Department of Health
1000 N.E. 10th
P.O. Box 53551
Oklahoma City, OK 73152

Oregon

Department of Human Resource,
   Health Division
800 N.E. Oregon Street
Portland, OR 97232

Pennsylvania

Department of Health
802 Health and Welfare Building
Harrisburg, PA 17120

Rhode Island

Department of Health
3 Capitol Hill
Providence, RI 02908

South Carolina

Health and Environmental Control
2600 Bull Street
Columbia, SC 29201

South Dakota

Department of Health
445 E. Capitol Avenue
Pierre, SD 57501

Tennessee

Department of Health
344 Cordell Hull
 Building
Nashville, TN 37247

Texas

Department of Health
1100 W. 49th Street
Austin, TX 78756

Utah

Department of Health
288 N. 1460 W.
Salt Lake City, UT 84116

Vermont

Department of Health
108 Cherry Street
P.O. Box 70
Burlington, VT 05402

Virginia

Department of Health
400 James Madison Building
109 Governor Street
Richmond, VA 23219

Washington

Department of Health
P.O. Box 47890
Olympia, WA 98504

West Virginia

Department of Health and Human
 Resources
Building 3
State Capitol Complex
Charleston, WV 25305

Wisconsin

Department of Health and Social
 Services
1 W. Wilson Street
Madison, WI 53703

Wyoming

Department of Health
Hathaway Building
Cheyenne, WY 82002

APPENDIX 2

State-by-State Listing of Long-Term Care Ombudsman Offices

Alabama

Commission on Aging
502 Washington Avenue
Montgomery, AL 36130

Alaska

Older Alaskans Ombudsman
2600 Denali Street, Suite 303
Anchorage, AK 99503

Arizona

Aging and Adult Administration
1400 W. Washington Street
P.O. Box 6123
Phoenix, AZ 85007

Arkansas

Office on Aging and Adult
    Services
Department of Human Services
Donaghey Building
7th and Main Streets
Little Rock, AR 72201

California

California Department on Aging
1020 19th Street
Sacramento, CA 95814

Colorado

Medical Care and Research
    Foundation
1565 Clarkson Street
Denver, CO 80218

Connecticut

Connecticut Department on Aging
175 Main Street
Hartford, CT 06106

Delaware

Division on Aging
Milford State Service Center
11-13 Church Avenue
Milford, DE 19963

District of Columbia

Legal Counsel for the Elderly
1331 H Street, N.W.
Washington, D.C. 20005

Florida

State Long Term Care Ombudsman
    Committee
Department of Health and
    Rehabilitative Services
Building #1
1317 Winewood Boulevard
Tallahassee, FL 32399

Georgia

Office on Aging
Department of Human Resources
878 Peachtree Street, N.E.
Atlanta, GA 30389

Hawaii

Hawaii Executive Office on Aging
335 Merchant Street
Honolulu, HI 96813

Idaho

Idaho Office on Aging
State House
Boise, ID 83720

Illinois

Department on Aging
421 East Capitol Avenue
Springfield, IL 62701

Indiana

Indiana Department of Aging and
Adult Community Services
Capitol Center, 251 North Illinois
Indianapolis, IN 46207

Iowa

Commission on the Aging
Jewett Building
916 Grand Avenue
Des Moines, IA 50319

Kansas

Department on Aging
610 West Tenth Street
Topeka, KS 66612

Kentucky

Division for Aging Services
275 East Main Street
Frankfort, KY 40601

Louisiana

Governor's Office of Elderly Affairs
P.O. Box 80374
4528 Bennington Avenue
Baton Rouge, LA 70898

Maine

Maine Committee on Aging
State House Station #11
Augusta, ME 04333

Maryland

Maryland Office on Aging
301 West Preston Street
Baltimore, MD 21201

Massachusetts

Massachusetts Executive Office of
Elder Affairs
38 Chauncy Street
Boston, MA 02111

Michigan

Citizens for Better Care
1627 East Kalamazoo
Lansing, MI 48917

Minnesota

Minnesota Board on Aging
Metro Square Building
7th and Robert Streets
St. Paul, MN 55101

Mississippi

Mississippi Council on Aging
301 West Pearl Street
Jackson, MS 39203

Missouri

Division on Aging
Department of Social Services
P.O. Box 1337
505 Missouri Boulevard
Jefferson City, MO 65102

Montana

Seniors' Office of Legal and
   Ombudsman Services
P.O. Box 232, Capitol Station
Helena, MT 59620

Nebraska

Department on Aging
P.O. Box 95044
301 Centennial Mall-South
Lincoln, NE 68509

Nevada

Division on Aging Services
Department of Human Resources
Kinkead Building
505 East King Street
Carson City, NV 89710

New Hampshire

New Hampshire State Council on
   Aging
Prescott Park
105 Loudon Road, Building #3
Concord, NH 03301

New Jersey

Office of the Ombudsman for the
   Institutionalized Elderly
CN 808
28 West State Street
Trenton, NJ 08625

New Mexico

State Agency on Aging
LaVilla Rivera Building
224 East Palace Avenue
Santa Fe, NM 87501

New York

Office for the Aging
Agency Building #2
Empire State Plaza
Albany, NY 12223

North Carolina

North Carolina Department of
   Human Resources
Division of Aging
Kirby Building
1985 Umpstead Drive
Raleigh, NC 27603

North Dakota

Aging Services Division
Department of Human Services
State Capitol Building
Bismarck, ND 58505

Ohio

Ohio Department on Aging
50 W. Broad Street
Columbus, OH 43215

Oklahoma

Special Unit on Aging
Department of Human Services
P.O. Box 25352
Oklahoma City, OK 73125

Oregon

Office of Long Term Care Ombudsman
2475 Lancaster Drive
Building B. #9
Salem, OR 97310

Pennsylvania

Department of Aging
Barto Building
231 State Street
Harrisburg, PA 17101

Rhode Island

Rhode Island Department of
  Elderly Affairs
79 Washington Street
Providence, RI 02903

South Carolina

Office of the Governor
Division of Ombudsman and
  Citizens' Services
1205 Pendleton Street
Columbia, SC 29203

South Dakota

Office of Adult Services and Aging
Department of Social Services
Richard F. Kneip Building
700 N. Illinois Street
Pierre, SD 57501

Tennessee

Commission on Aging
715 Tennessee Building
535 Church Street
Nashville, TN 37219

Texas

Texas Department on Aging
P.O. Box 12786 Capitol Station
Austin, TX 78704

Utah

Division of Aging and Adult Services
Department of Social Services
150 W. North Temple
Salt Lake City, UT 04103

Vermont

Vermont Office on Aging
103 South Main Street
Waterbury, VT 05676

Virginia

Department for the Aging
101 N. 14th Street
James Monroe Building
Richmond, VA 23219

Washington

Division of Audit
Department of Social and Health
  Services
MS OB-44-Y
Olympia, WA 98504

West Virginia

Commission on Aging
State Capitol Complex
Charleston, WV 25305

Wisconsin

Board on Aging and Long Term Care
819 North 6th
Milwaukee, WI 53203

Wyoming

Wyoming State Bar Association
900 8th Street
Wheatland, WY 82201

APPENDIX 3

State-by-State Listing of Departments of Insurance

Alabama

Department of Insurance
135 S. Union Street
Montgomery, AL 36130

Alaska

Division of Insurance
Department of Commerce and
 Economic Development
P.O. Box 110805
Juneau, AK 99811

Arizona

Department of Insurance
3030 N. Third Street
Phoenix, AZ 85012

Arkansas

Department of Insurance
Tower Building, Suite 400
1123 S. University
Little Rock, AR 72204

California

Department of Insurance
45 Freemont Street, 23rd Floor
San Francisco, CA 94105

Colorado

Division of Insurance
Department of Regulatory Agencies
1560 Broadway, Suite 850
Denver, CO 80204

Connecticut

Department of Insurance
P.O. Box 816
Hartford, CT 06142

Delaware

Department of Insurance
18 The Green
Dover, DE 19901

District of Columbia

Insurance Administration
Department of Consumer and
 Regulatory Affairs
613 C Street, N.W., Room 600
Washington, D.C. 20001

Florida

Department of Insurance
State Capitol, FL11
Tallahassee, FL 32399

Georgia

Office of Insurance Commissioner
704 West Tower
2 Martin Luther King, Jr., Drive
Atlanta, GA 30334

Hawaii

Division of Insurance
Department of Commerce and Consumer Affairs
101 Richards Street
Honolulu, HI 96813

Idaho

Department of Insurance
500 S. 10th
Boise, ID 83720

Illinois

Department of Insurance
320 W. Washington, 4th Floor
Springfield, IL 62767

Indiana

Department of Insurance
311 W. Washington Street, Suite 300
Indianapolis, IN 46204

Iowa

Insurance Division
Department of Commerce
Lucas State Office Building
Des Moines, IA 50319

Kansas

Department of Insurance
420 S.W. Ninth Street
Topeka, KS 66612

Kentucky

Department of Insurance
229 West Main Street
Frankfort, KY 40601

Louisiana

Department of Insurance
P.O. Box 94214
Baton Rouge, LA 70804

Maine

Bureau of Insurance
State House Station #34
Augusta, ME 04333

Maryland

Division of Insurance
Department of Licensing and
   Regulation
501 St. Paul Street
Baltimore, MD 21202

Massachusetts

Division of Insurance
Executive Office of Consumer Affairs
280 Friend Street
Boston, MA 02114

Michigan

Commissioner of Insurance
Department of Licensing and
   Regulation
P.O. Box 30220
Lansing, MI 48909

Minnesota

Department of Commerce
133 East Seventh Street
St. Paul, MN 55101

Mississippi

Department of Insurance
1804 Sillers Building
Jackson, MS 39201

Missouri

Department of Insurance
301 West High Street
P.O. Box 690
Jefferson City, MO 65102

Montana

Insurance Division
P.O. Box 4009
Helena, MT 59604

Nebraska

Department of Insurance
The Terminal Building, Suite 400
941 O Street
Lincoln, NE 68508

Nevada

Insurance Division
Department of Commerce
1665 Hot Springs Road
Carson City, NV 89710

New Hampshire

Insurance Department
169 Manchester Street
Concord, NH 03301

New Jersey

Department of Insurance
20 West State Street, CN 325
Trenton, NJ 08625

New Mexico

Department of Insurance
PERA Building, Room 428
Santa Fe, NM 87503

New York

Department of Insurance
Agency Building #1
Empire State Plaza
Albany, NY 12257

North Carolina

Department of Insurance
430 North Salisbury Street
Raleigh, NC 27603

North Dakota

Department of Insurance
State Capitol, 5th Floor
600 East Boulevard Avenue
Bismarck, ND 58505

Ohio

Department of Insurance
2100 Stella Court
Columbus, OH 43266

Oklahoma

Department of Insurance
408 Will Rogers Building
Oklahoma City, OK 73105

Oregon

Department of Consumer and
    Business Services
21 Labor and Industries Building
Salem, OR 97310

Pennsylvania

Department of Insurance
Strawberry Square, 13th Floor
Harrisburg, PA 17120

Rhode Island

Department of Insurance
233 Richmond Street, Suite 233
Providence, RI 02901

South Carolina

Department of Insurance
1612 Marion Street
Columbia, SC 29201

South Dakota

Department of Commerce and
  Regulations
910 East Sioux Avenue
Pierre, SD 57501

Tennessee

Department of Commerce and
  Insurance
500 James Robertson Parkway
Nashville, TN 37243

Texas

Board of Insurance
1110 San Jacinto Boulevard
Austin, TX 78701

Utah

State Insurance Department
3110 State Office Building
Salt Lake City, UT 84114

Vermont

Department of Banking, Insurance,
  and Securities
120 State Street
Montpelier, VT 05602

Virginia

State Corporation Commission
1220 Bank Street, 13th Floor
Richmond, VA 23219

Washington

Office of the Insurance
  Commissioners
Insurance Building
P.O. Box 40155
Olympia, WA 98504

West Virginia

Division of Insurance
2100 Washington Street, East
Charleston, WV 25305

Wisconsin

Office of Insurance Commissioner
123 West Washington Avenue
P.O. Box 7873
Madison, WI 53707

Wyoming

Department of Insurance
Herschler Building
Cheyenne, WY 82002

State-by-State Listing of Medical and Nursing Boards

Alabama

State Board of Nursing
RSA Plaza
770 Washington Avenue
Montgomery, AL 36130

State Board of Medical Examiners
848 Washington Avenue
Montgomery, AL 36104

Alaska

State Board of Nursing
3601 C Street
Anchorage, AK 99503

State Medical Board
3601 C Street
Anchorage, AK 99503

Arizona

State Board of Nursing
2001 West Camelback Road
Phoenix, AZ 85015

State Board of Medical Examiners
1651 East Morton
Phoenix, AZ 85020

Arkansas

State Board of Nursing
University Tower Building
1123 South University Avenue
Little Rock, AR 72204

State Medical Board
2100 Riverfront Drive
Harrisburg, AR 72202

California

State Board of Registered Nursing
P.O. Box 944210
Sacramento, CA 94244

State Medical Board
1426 Howe Avenue
Sacramento, CA 95825

Colorado

State Board of Nursing
1560 Broadway
Denver, CO 80202

State Board of Medical Examiners
1560 Broadway
Denver, CO 80202

Connecticut

State Board of Nursing
150 Washington Street
Hartford, CT 06106

Division of Medical Quality Assurance
150 Washington Street
Hartford, CT 06106

Delaware

State Board of Nursing
Margaret O'Neill Building
P.O. Box 1401
Dover, DE 19903

State Board of Medical Practice
Margaret O'Neill Building
P.O. Box 1401
Dover, DE 19903

District of Columbia

Board of Nursing
614 H Street, N.W.
Washington, D.C. 20001

Board of Medicine
605 G Street, N.W.
Lower Level
Washington, D.C. 20013

Florida

State Board of Nursing
111 Coast Line Drive, E.
Jacksonville, FL 32202

State Board of Medicine
1940 North Monroe Street
Northwood Centre
Tallahassee, FL 32399

Georgia

State Board of Nursing
166 Pryor Street, S.W.
Atlanta, GA 30303

State Board of Medical Examiners
166 Pryor Street, S.W.
Atlanta, GA 30303

Hawaii

State Board of Nursing
P.O. Box 3469
Honolulu, HI 96801

State Board of Medical Examiners
1010 Richards Street
Honolulu, HI 96813

Idaho

State Board of Nursing
280 North 8th Street
Boise, ID 83720

State Board of Medicine
State House Mall
280 North 8th Street
Boise, ID 83720

Illinois

Department of Professional
    Regulation, Nurse Section
320 West Washington Street
Springfield, IL 62786

Department of Professional
    Regulation, Medical Section
100 West Randolph Street
Chicago, IL 60601

Indiana

State Board of Nursing
1 American Square
P.O. Box 82067
Indianapolis, IN 46282

State Medical Licensing Board
402 West Washington
Indianapolis, IN 46204

Iowa

State Board of Nursing
State Capitol Complex
1223 East Court Avenue
Des Moines, IA 50319

State Board of Medical Examiners
State Capitol Complex
Executive Hills West
1209 East Court Avenue
Des Moines, IA 50319

Kansas

State Board of Nursing
Landon State Office Building
900 S.W. Jackson
Topeka, KS 66612

State Board of Healing Arts
235 S.W. Topeka Boulevard
Topeka, KS 66603

Kentucky

State Board of Nursing
312 Whittington Parkway
Louisville, KY 40222

Board of Medical Licensure
The Hurstbourne Office Park
310 Whittington Parkway
Louisville, KY 40222

Louisiana

State Board of Nursing
912 Pere Marquette Building
New Orleans, LA 70112

State Board of Medical Examiners
830 Union Street
New Orleans, LA 70112

Maine

State Board of Nursing
35 Anthony Avenue
State House Station
Augusta, ME 04333

State Board of Registration in
  Medicine
2 Bangor Street
State House Station
Augusta, ME 04333

Maryland

State Board of Nursing
4140 Patterson Avenue
Baltimore, MD 21215

State Board of Physician Quality
  Assurance
4201 Patterson Avenue
Baltimore, MD 21215

Massachusetts

State Board of Registration in
  Nursing
100 Cambridge Street
Boston, MA 02202

State Board of Registration in
  Medicine
Ten West Street
Boston, MA 02111

Michigan

State Board of Nursing
611 West Ottawa Street
P.O. Box 30018
Lansing, MI 48909

State Board of Medicine
611 West Ottawa Street
P.O. Box 30192
Lansing, MI 48909

Minnesota

State Board of Nursing
2700 University Avenue, W.
St. Paul, MN 55114

State Board of Medical Practice
2700 University Avenue, W.
St. Paul, MN 55114

Mississippi

State Board of Nursing
239 North Lamar Street
Jackson, MS 39201

State Board of Medical Licensure
2688-D Insurance Center Drive
Jackson, MS 39216

Missouri

State Board of Nursing
3605 Missouri Boulevard
P.O. Box 656
Jefferson City, MO 65102

State Board of Registration for the
  Healing Arts
3605 Missouri Boulevard
Jefferson City, MO 65102

Montana

State Board of Nursing
111 North Jackson
P.O. Box 200513
Arcade Building
Helena, MT 59620

State Board of Medical Examiners
111 North Jackson
P.O. Box 200513
Helena, MT 59620

Nebraska

State Board of Examiners in
  Medicine and Surgery
301 Centennial Mall, S.
P.O. Box 95007
Lincoln, NE 68509

Nevada

State Board of Nursing
1281 Terminal Way
Reno, NV 89502

State Board of Medical Examiners
1105 Terminal Way
Reno, NV 89502

New Hampshire

State Board of Nursing
Division of Public Health Services
6 Hazen Drive
Concord, NH 03301

State Board of Registration of
  Medicine
2 Industrial Park Drive
Concord, NH 03301

New Jersey

State Board of Nursing
124 Halsy Street
Newark, NH 07101

State Board of Medical Examiners
140 East Front Street
Trenton, NH 08608

New Mexico

State Board of Nursing
4206 Louisiana NE
Albuquerque, NM 87109

State Board of Medical Examiners
491 Old Santa Fe Trail
Lamy Building
P.O. Box 20001
Santa Fe, MN 87501

New York

State Board of Nursing
The Cultural Center
Albany, NY 12230

State Board of Medicine
Cultural Education Center
Empire State Plaza
Albany, NY 12230

North Carolina

State Board of Nursing
P.O. Box 2129
Raleigh, NC 27602

State Board of Medical Examiners
1203 Front Street
Raleigh, NC 27609

North Dakota

State Board of Nursing
919 South 7th Street
Bismarck, ND 58504

State Board of Medical Examiners
City Center Plaza
418 East Broadway Avenue
Bismarck, ND 58501

Ohio

State Board of Nursing
77 South High Street
Columbus, OH 43266

State Medical Board
77 South High Street
Columbus, OH 43266

Oklahoma

State Board of Nursing
2915 South Classen Boulevard
Oklahoma City, OK 73106

State Board of Medical Licensure
   and Supervision
5104 North Francis
Oklahoma City, OK 73118

Oregon

State Board of Nursing
800 N.E. Oregon Street
Portland, OR 97232

State Board of Medical Examiners
620 Crown Plaza
1500 S.W. First Avenue
Portland, OR 97201

Pennsylvania

State Board of Nursing
P.O. Box 2649
Harrisburg, PA 17105

State Board of Medicine
Transportation and Safety Building
Commonwealth and Forster Street
Harrisburg, PA 17105

Rhode Island

State Board of Nursing Education
  and Registration
3 Capitol Hill
Providence, RI 02908

State Board of Medical Licensure
  and Discipline
Cannon Building
3 Capitol Hill
Providence, RI 02908

South Carolina

State Board of Nursing
220 Executive Center Drive
Columbia, SC 29210

State Board of Medical Examiners
101 Executive Center Drive
Saluda Building
Columbia, SC 29210

South Dakota

State Board of Nursing
3307 South Lincoln
Sioux Falls, SD 57105

State Board of Medical and
  Osteopathic Examiners
1323 South Minnesota Avenue
Sioux Falls, SD 57105

Tennessee

State Board of Nursing
283 Plus Park Boulevard
Nashville, TN 37217

State Board of Medical Examiners
287 Plus Park Boulevard
Nashville, TN 37217

Texas

State Board of Nurse Examiners
9101 Burnet Road
Austin, TX 78758

State Board of Medical Examiners
1812 Centre Creek
Austin, TX 78714

Utah

State Board of Nursing
160 East 300 South
P.O. Box 45805
Salt Lake City, UT 84145

Physicians Licensing Board
Heber M. Wells Building
160 East 300 South
Salt Lake City, UT 84145

Vermont

State Board of Nursing Licensure
  and Regulation
109 State Street
Montpelier, VT 05609

State Board of Medical Practice
109 State Street
Montpelier, VT 05609

Virginia

State Board of Nursing
6606 West Broad Street
Richmond, VA 23230

State Board of Medicine
6606 West Broad Street
Richmond, VA 23230

Washington

State Board of Nursing
P.O. Box 47864
Olympia, WA 98504

State Medical Board
1300 S.E. Quince Street
P.O. Box 47866
Olympia, WA 98504

West Virginia

State Board of Examiners for
    Registered Professional
    Nurses
101 Dee Drive
Charleston, WV 25311

State Board of Medicine
101 Dee Drive
Charleston, WV 25311

Wisconsin

State Bureau of Health Service
    Professionals
1400 East Washington Avenue
P.O. Box 8935
Madison, WI 53708

Medical Examining Board
1400 East Washington Avenue
Madison, WI 53708

Wyoming

State Board of Nursing
Barrett Building
2301 Central Avenue
Cheyenne, WY 82002

State Board of Medicine
Barrett Building
2301 Central Avenue
Cheyenne, WY 82002

APPENDIX 5

Sample Voluntary Arbitration Agreement

1. I voluntarily agree to submit to arbitration any and all claims involving persons bound by this agreement (as set forth in Article 2 herein) whether those claims are brought in tort, contract, or otherwise. This includes, but is not limited to, suits for personal injury, actions to collect debts, or any kind of civil action.

2. I understand and agree that this Agreement binds me, my heirs, assigns, or personal representative and the undersigned physician, his/her professional corporation or partnership, if any, his/her employees, partners, heirs, assigns, or personal representative, and any consenting substitute physician. I also hereby consent to the intervention or joinder in the arbitration proceeding of all parties relevant to a full and complete settlement of any dispute arbitrated under this Agreement.

3. I agree to accept medical services from the undersigned physician and to pay for those services.

4. I understand that I do not have to sign this Agreement to receive the physician's services, and that if I do sign the Agreement and change my mind within 30 days of signing, then I may revoke this Agreement by giving written notice to the undersigned physician within that time stating my intention to withdraw from this Arbitration Agreement.

5. I agree to be bound by the State Arbitration Rules hereby incorporated into this Agreement.

6. I have read and understood this Agreement, including the Rules, and this writing makes up the entire Arbitration Agreement between me and the undersigned physician.

NOTICE: BY SIGNING THIS AGREEMENT YOU ARE CONSENTING TO HAVE ANY ISSUE OF MEDICAL MALPRACTICE DECIDED BY NEUTRAL ARBITRATION AND ARE WAIVING YOUR RIGHT TO A JURY OR COURT TRIAL.

Dated: _____   _____

Patient's Signature

Physician's Agreement to Arbitrate

In consideration of the above-named patient's promise to be bound by the Arbitration Agreement, I agree to be similarly bound by the terms of this Agreement as set forth above and in the Rules referred to herein.

Dated: _____   _____

Physician's Signature

APPENDIX 6

Sample Consent Form

Patient's Name: _____ Age: _____

Date: _____ Time: _____

Consent obtained at: _____
(i.e., hospital, physician's office)

1. I authorize the performance upon _____ of the following
(Myself or patient's name)

operation or procedure _____ to be performed at
(State nature and extent of operation)

_____ under the direction of Dr. _____

(Name of medical facility)   (Name of physician/surgeon)

and/or such associates and assistants as may be selected by him.

2. The nature and purpose of the operation referred to herein and the possible alternative methods of treatment have been explained to me by Dr. _____ to my satisfaction. No guarantee or assurance has

(Name of physician/surgeon)

been given by anyone as to the results that may be obtained.

3. I acknowledge that I have been afforded the opportunity to ask any questions with respect to the operation and any risks or complications thereto and to set forth, in the space provided below, any limitations or restrictions with respect

to this consent: _____

_____

4. I consent to the performance of operations, procedures, and treatments in addition to or different from those now contemplated as described above, whether or not arising from presently unforeseen conditions, which the above-named doctor or his or her associates or assistants may in their judgment consider necessary or advisable in my present illness.

5. I understand that anesthesia shall be administered during this operation under the direction of the responsible physician.

6. For the purpose of advancing medical education, I consent to the admittance of observers to the operating room.

7. I consent to the disposal by hospital authorities of any tissues or parts that may be removed.

I CERTIFY I HAVE READ AND FULLY UNDERSTAND THE ABOVE CONSENT, THAT THE EXPLANATIONS THEREIN REFERRED TO WERE MADE. THAT ALL BLANKS OR STATEMENTS REQUIRING INSERTION OR COMPLETION WERE FILLED IN, AND THAT INAPPLICABLE PARAGRAPHS, IF ANY, WERE STRICKEN BEFORE I SIGNED.

Signature of Patient: _____ Signature of Witness: _____

When a patient is a minor or incompetent to give consent:

Signature of person authorized to consent for patient: _____

Relationship to patient: _____

The foregoing consent was signed in my presence, and in my opinion the person did so freely with full knowledge and understanding.

Signature of Physician: _____ Signature of Witness: _____

APPENDIX 7

Listing of Advocacy Organizations by Disease

GENERAL INFORMATION

National Health Information Center   1-800-336-4797
National Information Center for Orphan Drugs and Rare
  Diseases   1-800-300-7469
National Women's Health Network   202-628-7814

LISTING BY DISEASE OR DISABILITY

AGING

National Institute on Aging Information Center   1-800-222-2225

AIDS/HIV

AIDS Clinical Trials Information Service   1-800-874-2572
Centers for Disease Control National AIDS Clearinghouse   1-800-458-5231
Centers for Disease Control National AIDS Hotline   1-800-342-AIDS
Project Inform HIV/AIDS Treatment Hotline   1-800-822-7422

ALCOHOL/DRUG ABUSE

ADCARE Hospital Hotline   1-800-ALCOHOL
Alcohol and Drug Helpline   1-800-821-4357
American Council on Alcoholism   1-800-527-5344
National Clearinghouse for Alcohol and Drug Information   1-800-729-6686
National Drug Information, Treatment and Referral Hotline   1-800-662-HELP
National Cocaine Hotline   1-800-262-2463

National Council on Alcoholism and Drug Dependence, Inc.   1-800-622-2255
Target Resource Center   1-800-366-6667

ALZHEIMER'S DISEASE

Alzheimer's Association   1-800-272-3900
Alzheimer's Disease Education and Referral Center   1-800-438-4380

ARTHRITIS

Arthritis Foundation Information Line   1-800-283-7800
National Arthritis and Musculoskeletal and Skin Diseases
    Information Clearinghouse   301-495-4484

CANCER

American Cancer Society Response Line   1-800-227-2345
Cancer Information Service   1-800-4-CANCER
National Marrow Donor Program   1-800-MARROW-2
Y-ME National Organization for Breast Cancer
    Information Support Program   1-800-221-2141

CANCER SUPPORT GROUPS

The Candlelighters Childhood Cancer Foundation
7910 Woodmont Ave., Suite 460
Bethesda, MD 20814
301-657-8401
This group provides a newsletter, list of local support groups, camps, bro-
chures, and information for siblings.

Chemocare
231 North Avenue West
Westfield, NJ 07090
908-233-1103 (in New Jersey)
1-800-55-CHEMO (elsewhere)
Chemocare offers free one-on-one counseling to patients undergoing cancer
treatment and their families. The organization has one satellite office in San
Diego and plans to open another office in Atlanta. Counseling is conducted
on the telephone when face-to-face meetings cannot be arranged.

American Cancer Society
1599 Clifton Road, NE
Atlanta, GA 30329
1-800-ACS-2345
The American Cancer Society provides a list of local support groups in your area upon request.

National Cancer Institute's Cancer Information Service
1-800-4 CANCER
In addition to providing information about local support groups, the operators at the NCI's Cancer Information Service can direct you to resources in your area that provide other services, such as transportation assistance and home-delivered meals.

CEREBRAL PALSY

United Cerebral Palsy Association   1-800-872-5827

CYSTIC FIBROSIS

Cystic Fibrosis Foundation   1-800-344-4823

DIABETES

American Diabetes Association   1-800-232-3472
Juvenile Diabetes Foundation International Hotline   1-800-223-1138
National Diabetes Information Clearinghouse   1-800-654-3327

DIGESTIVE DISEASE

National Digestive Diseases Information Clearinghouse   301-654-3810
Crohn's and Colitis Foundation of America, Inc.   1-800-932-2423

DISABILITIES

Clearinghouse on Disability Information   202-205-8241
National Information Center for Children and Youth with
  Disabilities   1-800-695-0285

National Rehabilitation Information Center   1-800-346-2742

Down's Syndrome

National Down Syndrome Congress   1-800-232-6372
National Down Syndrome Society Hotline   1-800-221-4602

Epilepsy

Epilepsy Foundation of America   1-800-332-1000

Heart Conditions

National Heart, Lung and Blood Institute Information Center   301-251-1222

Kidney and Urologic Disease

American Association of Kidney Patients   1-800-749-2257
American Foundation for Urologic Disease   1-800-242-2383
National Kidney and Urologic Diseases Information
    Clearinghouse   301-654-4415
National Kidney Foundation   1-800-622-9010
The Simon Foundation for Continence   1-800-237-4666

Learning Disorders

The Orton Dyslexia Society   1-800-222-3123

Liver Diseases

American Liver Foundation   1-800-223-0179

Lung Disease/Asthma/Allergy

Asthma and Allergy Foundation of America   1-800-727-8462
Asthma Information Hotline   1-800-822-2762

Lung Line National Jewish Center for Immunology and
    Respiratory Medicine   1-800-222-5864
National Institute of Allergy and Infectious Diseases   301-496-5717

Lupus

American Lupus Society   1-800-331-1802
Lupus Foundation of America   1-800-558-0121

Mental Health

Depression Awareness   1-800-421-4211
National Clearinghouse on Family Support and Children's
    Mental Health   1-800-628-1696
National Institute of Mental Health   301-443-4513

Multiple Sclerosis

National Multiple Sclerosis Society   1-800-344-4867

Paralysis and Spinal Cord Injury

American Heart Association Stroke Connection   1-800-553-6321
American Paralysis Association   1-800-225-0292
American Paralysis Association Spinal Cord Injury Hotline   1-800-526-3456
National Spinal Cord Injury Association   1-800-962-9629
National Stroke Association   1-800-STROKES

Parkinson's Disease

American Parkinson Disease Foundation   1-800-223-2732
National Parkinson Foundation, Inc.   1-800-327-4545
Parkinson's Education Program   1-800-344-7872

Sickle Cell Disease

National Association for Sickle Cell Disease   1-800-421-8453

SMOKING

Office on Smoking and Health at the Federal Centers for
Disease Control and Prevention   404-488-5708

SPEECH AND HEARING

American Speech-Language-Hearing Association   1-800-638-8255
Hear Now   1-800-648-4327
Hearing Helpline   1-800-327-9355

SUDDEN INFANT DEATH SYNDROME

American SIDS Institute   1-800-232-7437
National SIDS Resource Center   703-821-8955

APPENDIX 8

Sample Medical Information Bureau Notice and Authorization

TEXT OF MIB NOTICE

Information regarding your insurability will be treated as confidential. [Name of insurance company], or its reinsurer(s), may, however, make a brief report thereon to the Medical Information Bureau, a non-profit membership organization of life insurance companies, which operates an information exchange on behalf of its members. If you apply to another Bureau member company for life or health insurance coverage, or a claim for benefits is submitted to such a company, the Bureau, upon request, will supply such company with the information in its file. Upon receipt of a request from you, the Bureau will arrange disclosure of any information it may have in your file. If you question the accuracy of information in the Bureau's file, you may contact the Bureau and seek a correction in accordance with the procedures set forth in the Federal Fair Credit Reporting Act. The address of the Bureau's Information Office is Post Office Box 105, Essex Station, Boston, Massachusetts 02112, telephone number (617) 426-3660. [Name of insurance company], or its reinsurer(s), may also release information in its file to other life insurance companies to whom you apply for life or health insurance, or to whom a claim for benefits may be submitted.

TEXT OF MIB AUTHORIZATION

I hereby authorize any licensed physician, medical practitioner, hospital, clinic or other medical or medically related facility, insurance company, the Medical Information Bureau or other organization, institution or person, that has any record or knowledge of me or my health, to give to the [Name of insurance company], or its reinsurer(s) any such information.

APPENDIX 9

State-by-State Listing of Hospital Licensure Agencies

Alabama

Division of Licensure and
   Certification
Department of Public Health
434 Monroe Street
Montgomery, AL 36130

Alaska

Health Facilities Licensing and
   Certification
4796-6 Business Park Boulevard,
   Building H
Anchorage, AK 99503

Arizona

Office of Health Care Licensure
Department of Health Services
1647 East Morten Avenue
Phoenix, AZ 85020

Arkansas

Division of Health Facility Services
Department of Health
4815 W. Markham Street
Little Rock, AR 72205

California

Licensing and Certification
Department of Health Services
1800 3rd Street
Sacramento, CA 95814

Colorado

Health Facilities Division
Department of Health
4300 Cherry Creek Drive South
Denver, CO 80222

Connecticut

Licensing and Certification
Department of Health Services
150 Washington Street
Hartford, CT 06106

Delaware

Office of Health Facilities Licensing
   and Certification
Department of Health and Social
   Services
3000 Newport Gap Pike
Wilmington, DE 19808

District of Columbia

Service Facility Regulation
   Administration
614 H Street, N.W.
Washington, D.C. 20001

Florida

Office of Licensure and Certification
Department of Health and
   Rehabilitative Services
2727 Mahan Drive
Tallahassee, FL 32308

Georgia

Health Care Section, Office of
Regulatory Services
Department of Human Resources,
Public Health Division
878 Peachtree Street
Atlanta, GA 30309

Hawaii

Hospital and Medical Facilities
Branch, Licensing and
Certification
Department of Health
P.O. Box 3378
Honolulu, HI 96801

Idaho

Bureau of Facility Standards
Department of Health and Welfare
450 W. State Towers
Boise, ID 83720

Illinois

Division of Health Care Facilities
Department of Public Health
535 W. Jefferson Street
Springfield, IL 62761

Indiana

Division of Acute Care Services
State Board of Health
1330 W. Michigan Street
Indianapolis, IN 46206

Iowa

Division of Health Facilities
Department of Inspection and
Appeals
Lucas State Office Building
Des Moines, IA 50319

Kansas

Bureau of Adult and Child Care
Facilities
Department of Health and
Environment
900 S. W. Jackson
Topeka, KS 66612

Kentucky

Division of Licensing and Regulation
Department for Health Services
275 E. Main Street
Frankfort, KY 40601

Louisiana

Health Standards Section
Department of Health and Hospitals
P.O. Box 3767
Baton Rouge, LA 70821

Maine

Division of Licensing and
Certification
Department of Human Services
State House Station #11
Augusta, ME 04333

Maryland

Office of Licensing and Certification
Department of Health and Mental
Hygiene
4201 Patterson Avenue
Baltimore, MD 21215

Massachusetts

Division of Health Care Quality
Department of Public Health
10 West Street
Boston, MA 02111

Michigan

Bureau of Health Systems
Department of Public Health
3423 N. Logan
P.O. Box 30195
Lansing, MI 48909

Minnesota

Health Resources Division
Department of Health
393 North Dunlap Street
P.O. Box 64900
St. Paul, MN 55164

Mississippi

Division of Health Facilities
  Licensure and Certification
Department of Health
2688 Insurance Center Drive
Jackson, MS 39216

Missouri

Bureau of Hospital Licensing and
  Certification
Department of Health
P.O. Box 570
Jefferson City, MO 65102

Montana

Health Facilities Division
Department of Health and
  Environmental Sciences
Cogswell Building
Helena, MT 59620

Nebraska

Bureau of Health Facilities Standards
Department of Health
301 Centennial Mall, S.
P. O. Box 95007
Lincoln, NE 68509

Nevada

Bureau of Licensure and
  Certification
Department of Human Resources,
  Health Division
505 E. King Street
Carson City, NV 89710

New Hampshire

Bureau of Health Facilities
  Administration
Department of Health and Human
  Services
6 Hazen Drive
Concord, NH 03301

New Jersey

Licensing, Certification, and
  Standards
Department of Health
John Fitch Plaza, CN 367
Trenton, NJ 08625

New Mexico

Department of Health, Licensing and
  Certification Bureau
525 Camino de los Marquez
Santa Fe, NM 87501

New York

Bureau of Hospital Services
Office of Health Systems
  Management
Empire State Plaza
Albany, NY 12237

North Carolina

Division of Facility Services
Department of Human Resources
P.O. Box 29530
Raleigh, NC 27626

North Dakota

Health Resources Section
Department of Health
600 E. Boulevard Avenue
Bismarck, ND 58505

Ohio

Office of Resources Development
Department of Health
P.O. Box 118
Columbus, OH 43266

Oklahoma

Department of Health
1000 N.E. 10th
Oklahoma City, OK 73117

Oregon

Health Care Licensure and Certification
Department of Human Resource,
  Health Division
P.O. Box 14450
Portland, OR 97214

Pennsylvania

Division of Hospitals, Bureau of
  Quality Assurance
Health and Welfare Building
Harrisburg, PA 17120

Rhode Island

Department of Health
3 Capitol Hill
Providence, RI 02908

South Carolina

Division of Health Licensing
Health and Environmental Control
2600 Bull Street
Columbia, SC 29201

South Dakota

Licensure and Certification Program
Department of Health
445 E. Capitol Avenue
Pierre, SD 57501

Tennessee

Division of Health Care
  Facilities
Department of Health
283 Plus Park Boulevard
Nashville, TN 37247

Texas

Bureau of Licensing and
  Certification
Department of Health
1100 W. 49th Street
Austin, TX 78756

Utah

Bureau of Health Facility Licensure
Department of Health
P.O. Box 16990
Salt Lake City, UT 84116

Vermont

Medical Care Regulation Division
Department of Health
60 Main Street
Burlington, VT 05402

Virginia

Office of Health Facilities Regulation
Department of Health
3600 West Broad Street
Richmond, VA 23230

Washington

Office of Field Services
Department of Health
Target Plaza
2725 Harrison Avenue, N.W.
P.O. Box 7852
Olympia, WA 98504

West Virginia

Office of Health Facility Licensure
and Certification
Department of Health and Human
Resources
Building 3
State Capitol Complex
Charleston, WV 25305

Wisconsin

Bureau of Quality Compliance
Department of Health and Social
Services
1 W. Wilson Street
P.O. Box 309
Madison, WI 53701

Wyoming

Health Facilities Licensing
Department of Health
Hathaway Building
Cheyenne, WY 82002

APPENDIX 10

State Laws on Advance Medical Directives and Sample Directives

JURISDICTIONS THAT AUTHORIZE LIVING WILLS AND APPOINTMENT OF HEALTH CARE AGENT

Arizona
Arkansas
California
Colorado
Connecticut
Delaware
District of Columbia
Florida
Georgia
Hawaii
Idaho
Illinois
Indiana
Iowa
Kansas

Kentucky
Louisiana
Maine
Maryland
Minnesota
Mississippi
Missouri
Montana
Nebraska
Nevada
New Hampshire
New Jersey
New Mexico
North Carolina
North Dakota

Ohio
Oklahoma
Oregon
Pennsylvania
Rhode Island
South Carolina
South Dakota
Tennessee
Texas
Utah
Vermont
Virginia
Washington
West Virginia
Wisconsin
Wyoming

STATES THAT AUTHORIZE LIVING WILLS ONLY

Alabama
Alaska

STATES THAT AUTHORIZE APPOINTMENT OF HEALTH CARE AGENT ONLY

Massachusetts
Michigan
New York

SAMPLE LIVING WILL

I, _____, being of sound mind, voluntarily make this statement concerning my medical treatment preferences. This statement is to be followed if I become permanently unable to make or communicate decisions regarding my medical treatment and interventions that may be employed to prolong my life.

I direct my physicians and all medical personnel responsible for my care to withhold or withdraw all life-sustaining procedures if I am diagnosed with any of the following conditions:

a. A terminal illness that is expected to cause my death within six (6) months.

b. Irreversible brain damage such that I will never regain decision-making capacity.

c. Incurable disease, injury, or illness with no reasonable expectation of recovery.

I further direct my physicians and all medical personnel responsible for my care to administer pain-relieving treatments and measures so that I will be afforded maximum comfort and relief.

I make this statement after careful reflection and contemplation, and as a final expression of my legal right to refuse unwanted medical treatment. It is my intention that this directive be honored by my family and physicians without judicial intervention.

I reserve the right to revoke this directive at any time, either by a written notice of revocation or in any other manner. No physician, hospital, or other health care provider who relies on this directive without actual knowledge of revocation shall bear any liability to myself, my estate, or any other person. If not revoked, this directive shall remain in effect indefinitely.

This directive shall not in any way limit the powers or authority I have given to any health care agent or surrogate, or alternate or successor health care agent or surrogate.

_____   _____
            Date   Patient's Signature

[Witness and/or notary may be required depending on state law.]

[NOTE: This sample directive is included for illustrative purposes only. It should not be relied on without the advice of a knowledgeable professional.]

SAMPLE DESIGNATION OF HEALTH CARE AGENT

I hereby designate ————————, residing at ————————
————————————, telephone number ———————,
to serve as my agent for the purpose of making medical treatment decisions on
my behalf in the event I become unable to make and communicate those decisions for myself.

If the person appointed above is unable, unwilling, or unavailable to act as
my health care agent, I hereby designate ————————, residing at
————————————————————,
telephone number ————————, as my substitute or alternative health
care agent.

I instruct my agent to make health care decisions in accordance with my
wishes as those are known to him or her and the following optional statement
of instructions: ————————————————————

This document, if not revoked by me, shall remain in effect indefinitely.

Date: ———————————— Signed: ————————————

Witness: ——————————— Witness: ————————————

[NOTE: This sample designation is included for illustrative purposes only. It
should not be relied on without the advice of a knowledgeable professional.]

Notes

1. "New York State Malpractice Study: Harvard Medical Practice Report," published in book form, *A Measure of Malpractice,* by Dr. Howard Hiatt, et. al. (Harvard University Press, 1993).
2. *Medication Error Study,* Physician Insurers Association of America, 1130 Connecticut Avenue, NW, Washington, D.C. 20036 (June 1993).
3. "Incidence of Adverse Drug Events and Potential Adverse Drug Events: implications for prevention," by David W. Bates, el al., *The Journal of the American Medical Association* (July 5, 1995).
4. *Medicine on Trial: The appalling story of ineptitude, malfeasance, neglect, and arrogance,* by Charles Inlander (New York: Prentice Hall Press, 1988).
5. For more information on unnecessary Caesarean sections, contact the International Caesarean Awareness Network (formerly the Caesarean Prevention Movement), P.O. Box 152, Syracuse, New York 13210; telephone number 315-424-1942.
6. "Alternatives to Hysterectomy: Bench to Bedside." Conference sponsored by the National Institutes of Health (May 23–24, 1995). Articles from the conference published in *Research Reports from the National Institute of Child Health and Human Development,* American College of Obstetricians and Gynecologists newsletter (October 1994).
7. "Breast Cancer Leads Lawsuits," Associated Press, *Newsday,* June 4, 1995, A19.
8. In Milwaukee, a grand jury returned a homicide indictment against a medical laboratory for misreading the Pap smears of two women who later died of cervical cancer. "Medical Laboratory Faces Charges in Cancer Deaths," by Gina Kolata, *The New York Times,* April 13, 1995, A16.

9. *Cancer at a Crossroad,* National Cancer Institute (1994).
10. "Cancer Care at HMOs: Do Limits Hurt," by Gina Kolata, *The New York Times,* October 26, 1994, C11.
11. Ibid.
12. "Outcomes of Patients with Hypertension and Non-insulin Dependant Diabetes Mellitus Treated by Different Systems and Specialties: Results from the Medical Outcomes Study," by Dr. Sheldon Greenfield, et. al., *The Journal of the American Medical Association* 274 143b (November 8, 1995).
13. "Stage of Cancer at Diagnosis for Medicare HMO and Fee-for-service Enrollees," by George Riley, et al., *American Journal of Public Health* 84 (October 1994).
14. "Cancer Care at HMOs: Do Limits Hurt," by Gina Kolata, *The New York Times,* October 26, 1994, C11.
15. "Check-Up for Hospitals," by David Zinman, *Newsday,* January 10, 1995, B23.
16. Ibid.
17. "People Want More Information for Health Choices, Survey Finds," by Milt Freudenheim, *The New York Times,* September 17, 1995, A38.
18. Ibid.
19. In 1994, the New York Department of Health stopped publishing the names of doctors who perform the fewest bypass operations. While acknowledging the correlation between low volume and high mortality in open-heart surgery, health officials defended their decision to withhold this information on the grounds that the numbers are too small to be statistically reliable. Consumer advocates countered that patients have a right to know the identity of heart surgeons who consistently do the poorest work.
20. Ibid.
21. "Report Cards on Cardiac Surgeons: Assessing New York State's approach," by Jesse Green, and Neil Wintfeld, *The New England Journal of Medicine* 332 1229 (May 4, 1995).
22. "Death-Rate Rankings Shake New York Cardiac Surgeons," by Elizabeth Bumiller, *The New York Times,* September 6, 1995. A1.
23. "At Utah Hospital, Innovative Way to Track Medical Quality," by Joel Brinkley, *The New York Times,* March 31, 1994, B8.
24. *Usefulness and Impact of National Practitioners Data Bank Reports,* Office of Inspector General, No. OE1-01-94-00030 (April 19, 1995).
25. *Annual Statistical Release,* Federation of State Medical Boards, 400 Fuller Wiser Road, Euless, TX 76039 (April 5, 1995).
26. "More Doctors Face Prosecution," by Thomas Maier, *Newsday,* April 18, 1995, A35.
27. "Why Do People Sue Doctors? A Study of Patients and Relatives Taking Legal Action," by Charles Vincent, et al., *The Lancet* 343 1609 (June 25, 1994).
28. *Medical Malpractice, A Framework for Action: Report to Congressional Requesters,* U.S. General Accounting Office (1987).

29. *Economic Implications of Rising Health Care Costs,* U.S. Congressional Budget Office (October 1992).
30. "Health Care Reform: Don't Tamper with the Legal System," by Andrew J. Simons, *Nassau Lawyer,* April 1993, 24.
31. *Estimating the Costs of Defensive Medicine,* Lewin-VH1, prepared for MMI Companies (January 1993).
32. *Self-Dealing for Ancillary Medical Services: Impact on the delivery of services,* by Dr. Mark Cooper, The Consumer Federation of America (June 8, 1989). The findings of the federation have been confirmed by at least five studies published in *The New England Journal of Medicine* and *Journal of the American Medical Association.* Recently the practice of self-referrals has become the subject of regulation.
33. *Defensive Medicine and Medical Malpractice,* U.S. Congress: Office of Technology Assessment (July 1994).
34. 1990 study conducted by the General Accounting Office.
35. "The Support Prognostic Model: The study to understand prognoses and preferences for outcomes and risks of treatments," by Dr. William Knaus, *American College of Physicians* 122 191 (February 1995). See also, "Program Predicts Life Expectancy for the Sick," by Jamie Talan, *Newsday,* February 14, 1995, B31.
36. *In re Yetter,* 62 Pa D & C2d 619 (CP Northhampton Co. 1973).
37. *In the Matter of Harvey "U",* 116 AD2d 351, 501 NYS2d 920 (1986).
38. "Clinical Trials: Why participate," *HealthFacts* 17 1 (January 1992).
39. "Teen Surveys Vs. Parental Consent," by Earl Lane, *Newsday,* April 11, 1995, B29.
40. *Evaluation of Human Subject Protections in Schizophrenia Research Conducted by the University of California Los Angeles* from the Office for Protection From Research Risks, Division of Human Subject Protections, National Institutes of Health (May 11, 1994).
41. The Department of Health and Human Services (DHHS) and Food and Drug Administration (FDA) regulations only permit waiver of informed consent under limited circumstances, and the criteria of the two agencies differ. Critics charge that neither set of regulations is workable when applied to resuscitation research. Critics charge that the DHHS regulations are unworkable when applied to resuscitation research because they require that the research involve "no more than minimal risk to the subjects." Experimental resuscitation research does not meet the government's definition of minimal risk.

    The FDA's regulations are also problematic when applied to resuscitation research because they allow waiver only where no approved therapy "provides an equal or greater likelihood of saving the life of the subject." The relative effectiveness of experimental resuscitation techniques and standard therapies is often unknown.

42. "Consensus on Ethics in Research is Elusive," by Philip J. Hilts, *The New York Times*, January 15, 1995, 24.

43. *Code of Medical Ethics: Current Opinions with Annotations*, by the Council on Ethical and Judicial Affairs, (Chicago: American Medical Association: 1992).

44. *Harris v. Thigpen*, 941 F2d 1495 (11th Cir 1991).

45. "Tests to Assess Risks for Cancer Raising Questions," by Gina Kolata, *The New York Times*, March 27, 1995, A1.

46. *Genetic Testing for Children and Adolescents: Who decides?*, by Dr. Dorothy C. Wertz, *Journal of the American Medical Association* 272 875 (September 21, 1994).

47. "Should Children be Told if Genes Predict Illness?" by Gina Kolata, *The New York Times*, September 26, 1994, A1.

48. "Screening and Informed Consent," by John M. Lee, *The New England Journal of Medicine*, 328 438 (February 11, 1993).

49. Some states make exceptions for mental health, substance abuse treatment, and reproductive health.

50. *Consent and Confidentiality in the Health Care of Children and Adolescents: A Legal Guide*, by J.M. Morrissey, et. al (New York: Free Press, 1986).

51. "Treating Adolescents: Legal and ethical considerations," by A. English, *Medical Clinics of North America* 74 1097 (1990).

52. "Girl Flees After Clash of Cultures on Illness," Special to *The New York Times*, *The New York Times*, November 12, 1994, 8.

53. "Debating Rights of Young Patients," by Gail B. Slap and Martha M. Jablow, *The New York Times*, November 11, 1994, C1.

54. American Academy of Child and Adolescent Psychiatry Position Statement: Drug and alcohol screening, *AACAP Newsletter*, Summer 1991, 31–32.

55. *Thornburgh v. American College of Obstetricians and Gynecologists*, 476 US 747 (1986).

56. *Planned Parenthood v. Casey*, 112 S.Ct. 2791 (1992).

57. *Roe v. Wade*, 410 US 113 (1973); *Doe v. Bolton*, 410 US 179 (1973).

58. See, for example, *Webster v. Reproductive Health Services*, 109 S.Ct. 3040 (1989).

59. For a critique of the privacy act, see "Privacy, Government Information, and Technology," by Priscilla Regan, *Public Administration Review* 46 629 (November–December 1986).

60. *In re Application of Hershey Medical Center*, 595 A2d 1290 (PA Superior Ct. 1991).

61. *In re Application of Hershey Medical Center*, 535 PA 9 (1993).

62. *Whalen v. Roe*, 429 US 589 (1977).

63. For a more in-depth discussion, see "The Constitutional Protection of Information Privacy," by F.S. Chlapowski, *Boston University Law Review* 133 (1991).

64. *United States v. Westinghouse*, 638 F2d 570 (3rd Cir 1980).

65. "Court Backs Privacy Right Over HIV," by Mary B. W. Tabor, *The New York Times*, February 1, 1994, B3.

66. See, for example, *Rasmussen v. South Florida Blood Services Inc.*, 500 S2d 533 (Fla. 1987) and *Soroka v. Dayton Hudson Corp.*, 1 Cal Rptr 2d 77 (1991).

67. *Privacy in America*, by David F. Linowes (Urbana: University of Illinois Press, 1989).

68. *Medical Monitoring and Screening in the Workplace: Results of a Survey—Background Paper*, U.S. Congress, Office Of Technology Assessment (Washington, D.C.: Government Printing Office, October 1991).

69. "Patients' Records are Treasure Trove for Budding Industry," by Michael W. Miller, *The Wall Street Journal*, February 27, 1992.

70. The case, *Stone v. Stow*, is discussed in "Matter of Privacy," by Jesse Vivian, *Drug Topics* 136 70 (1992).

71. This legal requirement is contained in the National Association of Insurance Commissioner's Insurance Information and Privacy Protection Model Act, which is law in at least twelve states and is voluntarily followed in all states where the insurers do business.

72. Nonmedical information (e.g., lifestyle information) in MIB files will be sent directly to the consumer. Sometimes decoded medical information will only be sent to a physician designated by the consumer.

73. *Health Information Privacy Survey*, Louis Harris and Associates, Westin A.F., Equifax Inc. (Atlanta, Georgia, 1993).

74. "Privacy Rules for DNA Databanks: Protecting coded 'future diaries,' " by George J. Annas, *Journal of the American Medical Association* 270 2346 (November 17, 1993).

75. *Health Care Reform: Report Cards are useful but Significant Issues Need to be Addressed*, U.S. General Accounting Office, Report #HEHS-94-219 (September 29, 1994).

76. *Health Data in the Information Age: Use, Disclosure, and Privacy*, edited by M. S. Donaldson and R. N. Lohr (Institute of Medicine, Washington, DC: National Academy Press; 1994). The report is available from the National Academy Press, telephone (202) 334-3313 or (800) 624-6242.

77. Mont. Code Ann §50-16-501.

78. Wash WRCA §70.02.005.

79. *Vernonia School District v. Acton*, U.S. Supreme Court Docket Number 94-590.

80. The Americans with Disabilities Act allows drug testing so long as the employer does not discriminate against an "otherwise qualified" person with a disability. A person who is currently engaged in the illegal use of drugs is not "otherwise qualified." Drug tests can be used to establish current illegal use of drugs.

81. "Confidential Health Services for Adolescents," *Journal of the American Medical Association* 269 1420 (March 17, 1993).

82. "Factors Affecting Adolescents' Use of Family Planning Clinics," by M. Chamie, S. Eisman, M.T. Orr, A. Torres, *Family Planning Perspective* 14 126 (1982).

83. For the American Medical Association's National Adolescent Health Coalition's recommendations on confidential health services for adolescents, see

Policy Compendium on Confidential Health Services for Adolescents, edited by J. Gans, (Chicago: American Medical Association National Coalition on Adolescent Health, 1993).

84. See *Confidential Health Services for Adolecents, sup.*
85. House Committee on Government Operations, *Equal Access to Health Care: Patient Dumping,* 100th Cong. 2d sess., H. Rep. 100-531, 1988, 5–7.
86. *Update in Patient Dumping Violations: 91 hospitals named in 1993 and first quarter of 1994,* by Dr. Sidney M. Wolfe, and Joan J. D. Stieber, MSW, Public Citizen's Health Research Group (October 1994).
87. If you would like the names of hospitals that have adopted flexible visiting policies and provide living-in accommodations to meet the special needs of hospitalized children, contact Children in Hospitals, Federation for Children with Special Needs, 95 Berkeley Street, Suite 104, Boston, MA 02116; telephone number 617-482-2915.
88. "The relation between the volume of coronary angioplasty procedures at hospitals treating Medicare beneficiaries and short-term mortality," by Jollis, et. al. *The New England Journal of Medicine* 331 1625 (December 15, 1994).
89. Ibid.
90. If you would like information about the treatment of pain, you can order the free publication *Acute Pain Management, A Patient's Guide* (AHCPR Publication No. 92-0021) from the Agency for Health Care Policy and Research (AHCPR) Publications Clearinghouse. AHCPR can be reached by writing to P.O. Box 8547, Silver Spring, MD 20907, or calling 1-800-358-9295. To order *Cancer Pain Guidelines: Patient Guide,* call the National Cancer Information Service at 1-800-4-CANCER and request AHCPR Publication No. 94-0595.
91. *Nursing Home Use After 65 in the U.S.: Differences and remaining lifetime use among subgroups and states,* Federal Agency for Health Policy and Research, Publication No. 91-0047 (1991).
92. U.S. Senate Committee on Finance, *Improving Quality Care in Nursing Homes: Hearing before the Subcommittee on Health for Families and the Uninsured of the Committee on Finance,* 101st Cong. 2d session, Wyoming, MI (28 August 1990).
93. *Smith v. Heckler,* 747 F2d 582 (10th Cir 1984).
94. "Aging and Health: Effects of the Sense of Control," by Rodin, *Science* 233 1271 (September 1986).
95. H.R. 391(l), 100th Cong., 1st sess., 472.
96. See, for example, *Clay County Manor, Inc. v. Luna, Commissioner, Department of Health and Environment, State of Tennessee,* No. 3-89-0608 (M.D. Tenn., filed Apr. 26, 1990), 24 Clearinghouse Review 254 (July 1990); *Roberson v. Wood,* 464 F. Supp. 983 (E.D.III. 1979); *Berry v. First Healthcare Corp.,* CCH Medicare/Medicaid, Paragraph 28,693 (D.N.H. October 26, 1977), 11 Clearinghouse Review 581 (October 1977).
97. H.R. 391(l), 100th Cong., 1st sess., 452.

98. If you are working with a local ombudsman and are not getting results, contact the state long-term care ombudsman for assistance.

99. "Tying Down the Elderly," by Lois K. Evans et al. *Journal of the American Geriatrics Society*, 37 65 (1989).

100. "Mechanical Restraint Use and Fall-related Injuries Among Residents of Skilled Nursing Facilities," by Dr. Mary E. Tinetti, *Annals of Internal Medicine* 16 369 (March 1992).

101. "The Fear of Liability and the Use of Restraints in Nursing Homes," by Sandra H. Johnson, *Law, Medicine & Health Care* 18 263 (Fall 1990); "Legal Issues Involved in the Use of Restraints: Analyzing the risk," by Alan R. Hunt, published in *Untie the Elderly: Quality Care Without Restraints* (U.S. Senate Special Committee on Aging, Senate Committee Print No. 101-90, December 4, 1989).

102. "Nursing Home Restraints and Legal Liability: Merging the standard of care and industry practice," by Marshall B. Kapp, JD MPH, *The Journal of Legal Medicine* 13 1 (1992).

103. *Nursing Home Residents Rights: Has the administration set a land mine for the landmark OBRA 1987 Nursing Home Reform Law,* Subcommittee on Aging, Senate Committee on Labor and Human Resources (June 13, 1991); Impact of Urinary Incontinence on Health-Care Costs, by Teh-wei Hu, *Journal of the American Geriatrics Society* 38 293 (March 1990).

104. "For the Frail and the Elderly, Restraints are often Deathtraps," by Joe Rigert et al., *Minneapolis Star-Tribute*, December 2, 1990, 1A.

105. Interpretive Guidelines, State Operations Manual, Department of Health and Human Services (Transmittal No. 250, April 1992).

106. "The Nursing Home Reform Law: Issues for Litigation," by Toby Edelman, *Clearinghouse Review* 24 545 (October 1990).

107. "The Care of Elderly Patients with Hip Fractures: Changes Since Implementation of the Prospective Payment System," by J.F. Fitzgerald, P.S. Moore, and R.S. Dittus, *The New England Journal of Medicine* 319 1392 (November 24, 1988).

108. *Fox v. Bowen*, CCH Medicare/Medicaid, Paragraph 39, 374, H-78-541 (J.A.C.), April 23, 1986.

109. *Nursing Home Utilization by Current Residents: United States, 1985,* by Esther Hing, for the U.S. Department of Health and Human Services, Public Health Service, Centers for Disease Control, National Center for Health Statistics (Superintendent of Documents, 1989).

110. "Transfer and Discharge of Nursing Home Residents," by Gershuny and Hirsh, *Medical Trial Techniques Quarterly* 477 (1980); "Liberty from Transfer Trauma: A fundamental life and liberty interest," by Colette I. Hughes, *Hastings Constitutional Law Quarterly* 9 429 (1982).

111. "Protecting Nursing home Residents, Tort Actions Are One Way," by P. Nemore, *Trial* 21 54 (December 1985).

112. See *Berry v. First Healthcare Corp.*, sup; *Fuzie v. Manor Care, Inc.*, 461 F. Supp. 689 (N.D. Ohio 1977).

113. The danger of retaliation is minimized by bringing a class action. A class action may be available when the alleged illegal activity has affected more than one resident. In a class action, a group of similarly situated residents join together in a single lawsuit against the facility. See "Protecting the Identity of Nursing Home Residents in Litigation," *The Nursing Home Law Letter*, no. 82 (Mar. 1984). This publication is available from the National Senior Citizens Law Center, 1815 H Street, NW. Suite 700, Washington, D.C. 20006; telephone number 202-887-5280.

114. "Nursing Home Abuses as Uniform Trade Practices," by Horvath and Nemore, *Clearinghouse Review* 20 801 (1986).

115. *Cruzan v. Director, Missouri Department of Health*, 497 U.S. 261 (1990).

116. The witnesses had not come forward earlier because they had known Nancy by her married name, and had not realized she was the same person until the case moved into the national media. "Nancy Beth Cruzan, 1957–1990," *Society for the Right to Die Newsletter* 10 (Spring 1991).

117. "Withholding Care from Patients: Boston Case Asks, Who Decides?" by Gina Kolata, *The New York Times*, April 3, 1995, A1; "Court Ruling Limits Rights of Patients," by Gina Kolata, *The New York Times*, April 22, 1995, 6.

118. "Comfort Care for Terminally Ill Patients: The Appropriate Use of Nutrition and Hydration," by Robert M. McCann, et al., *Journal of the American Medical Association*, 272 1263 (October 26, 1994).

119. *Matter of Westchester County Medical Society (O'Connor)*, 72 NY2d 517 (1988).

120. "Flaws Surfacing in Use of Advance Directives," by Brian McCormick, *American Medical News* 35 1 (August 24, 1995).

121. "A Controlled Trial to Improve Care for Seriously Ill Hospitalized Patients," The SUPPORT principal investigators, *Journal of the American Medical Association* 274 1591 (November 22, 1995).

122. Ibid.

123. "The Aged Reject CPR Use," Associated Press, *The New York Times*, March 1, 1994, C6.

124. "Use of the Medical Futility Rationale in Do-Not-Attempt-Resuscitation Orders," by J. Randall Curtis, et. al., *Journal of the American Medical Association*, 273 124 (January 11, 1995).

125. "Uncharted Law for a Man Between Life and Death," by Michael deCourcy Hinds, *The New York Times*, June 6, 1994, B9.

126. "Family Wins Right to End Son's Ordeal," Associated Press, *The New York Times*, October 18, 1994, A20.

127. "Decisions Near the End of Life," *Journal of the American Medical Association* 267 2229 (April 22, 1992).

128. You can reach Compassion in Dying by writing to P.O. Box 75295, Seattle, WA 98125-0295 or calling 206-624-2775.

129. *Final Exit: The Practicalities of Self-Deliverance and Assisted Suicide for the Dying*, by Derek Humphrey (Secaucus, New Jersey: Hemlock Society, 1991).

130. "Death and Dignity: A Case of Individualized Decision-Making," *The New England Journal of Medicine* 324 691 (March 7, 1991).

131. Ibid.

132. *Compassion in Dying v. State of Washington*, 1994 WL 174250 (W.D. Wash., May 3, 1994).

133. *Compassion in Dying v. Washington*, Docket Number 94-35534 (March 1995).

134. Interestingly, the appellate ruling was written by a judge who was an anti-abortion legal theoretician and Catholic scholar before he was appointed to the bench by President Ronald Reagan in 1986.

135. *Hobbins v. Attorney General*, 1994 Mich App LEXIS 232 (Mich. App., May 10, 1994).

136. *Quill, et. al. v. Vacco, et. al.*, Second Circuit Court of Appeals, Docket Number 95-7028.

137. The law under which Dr. Kevorkian was acquitted was only a temporary measure and was subsequently repealed.

138. Some jurors had also been convinced by a less central argument made by the defense that Mr. Hyde's death had not taken place where the prosecution alleged. Dr. Kevorkian had been charged by city of Detroit authorities with assisting the suicide in the doctor's van in Belle Isle, a city park. Defense counsel argued to the jury that the suicide had actually taken place in a parking space behind Dr. Kevorkian's apartment in Oakland County, and that Dr. Kevorkian had only later driven the van to Belle Isle to surrender to the police. Defense counsel argued that the legal doctrine of double jeopardy prevented Oakland County prosecutors from retrying Dr. Kevorkian on the charges already filed by city prosecutors.

139. "Granting Father's Wish, or Manslaughter?", by Esther B. Fein, *The New York Times*, October 28, 1994, A1.

Index